DENTAL INTE
FIRST EDITION

A comprehensive guide to
DCT & ST interview skills

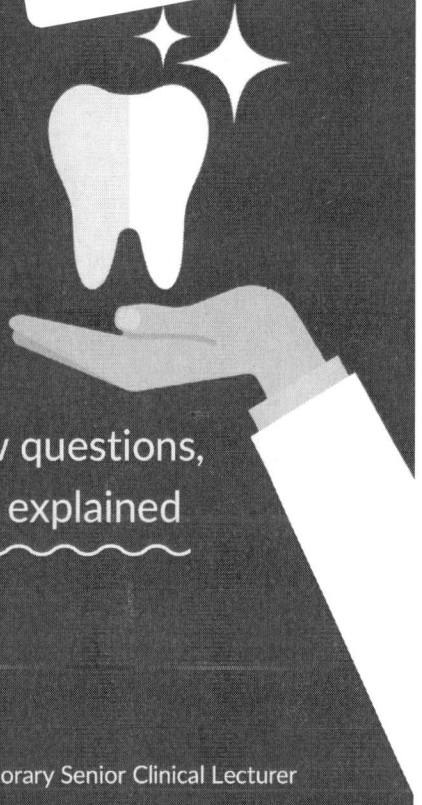

Over 120 medical interview questions,
techniques and NHS topics explained

Written by:
Ross Elledge MMEd FRCS (OMFS)
Consultant Oral and Maxillofacial Surgeon / Honorary Senior Clinical Lecturer

Olivier Picard BSc (Hons) MSc

Published by ISC Medical
Tel: 0203 507 0001 – Email: enquiries@iscmedical.co.uk

First Edition

Published by ISC Medical
Tel: 0203 507 0001 – Email: enquiries@iscmedical.co.uk

First Edition
ISBN13: 978-1-905812-25-7

Printed: March 2020

A catalogue record for this book is available from the British Library.

Printed in the United Kingdom by:
Optichrome Ltd, Maybury Road, Woking, Surrey GU21 5HX

The authors have, as far as possible, taken care to ensure that the information given in this text is accurate and up to date at the time of publication. The information within this text is intended as a revision aid for the purpose of medical interviews. It is not intended, nor should it be used, as a medical reference for the management of patients or their conditions. Readers are strongly advised to confirm that the information with regard to specific patient management complies with current legislation, guidelines and local protocols.

Contents

Preface

Dental specialty training is becoming increasingly competitive. To take oral surgery training as one example, in the first round of recruitment of 2019, there were around 120 applicants for eight posts. Many medical specialties don't even come close to such cut-throat competition ratios.

With a changing workforce and a growing trend across the board for provision of care in primary care, competition for consultant roles is fiercer still. The days of an informal "chat" and phone calls of recommendation from current employers are gone. The need for fairness, transparency and reproducibility has led to the introduction of the selection centre, with multiple stations, multiple assessors and multiple scoring opportunities against clinical skills and "softer skills" through assessment modalities, including objective structured clinical examinations (OSCEs), portfolio assessments and situational judgement tests (SJTs).

Know yourself well

Think about why you want this opportunity to train in a particular dental specialty. The people who interview and assess you are looking at you as a prospective member of their "club" in the smaller dental specialties and, as such, are looking for shared enthusiasm. Above and beyond that, however, they are looking for aptitude and a sense of the job being "tried and tested". They want to know that you have an understanding of what the job will involve beyond training, that you have form as well as aspiration, and that you have a solid groundwork to build upon in terms of core skills.

If you are applying for a specialty training programme in orthodontics, it would make sense to have some fundamental experience in adjusting removable appliances, debonding fixed appliances, etc, as core skills developed to "hit the ground running" in your higher training. Complementary experience in allied specialties that may interface with orthodontics (e.g. oral and maxillofacial surgery, paediatric dentistry) would also pay dividends in making you an effective member of a multidisciplinary team. In short, there is no bad experience; there are only bad ways of selling the lessons learnt.

Learn, understand and apply key communication frameworks

Many candidates wrongly assume that lack of knowledge will let them down in the interview process. In fact, knowledge makes up a relatively small component of what is assessed in interviews for training positions; arguably, most consultants would arguably prefer a trainee who is good "raw material" and able to be moulded throughout training. Knowledge can be taught and acquired. Attitude and aptitude are more important, and these can be demonstrated through mature, enthusiastic and confident responses to questions.

You will need frameworks, structures and checklists to build confident and well-structured answers to interview questions, using experience and skills that you already have at your disposal. The aim of this book is to apply techniques in order to structure answers and illustrate these structures with personal examples, helping you present well-thought-out and dynamic, but still natural, answers.

Practise, practise, practise

Natural answers paradoxically come from practice. This does not mean learning answers *verbatim*, but rather recognising that, despite the possibility of hundreds of different questions being fired at you in an interview, many will return to the same themes. By reading this book, you will quickly come to the realisation that, although you could be asked hundreds of questions, you will get back to the same handful of themes and communication techniques. Therefore, do not try to learn answers by heart. Instead, concentrate on developing good personal knowledge of the topics that are being addressed and the techniques required to organise your answers. This will give you greater flexibility and a definite ability to cope with pretty much any question.

Good luck with your preparation.

Ross Elledge and Olivier Picard

How to use this book

This book has been written in a modular fashion so that you can read it in many different ways.

If you have plenty of time to prepare
If you have time, you may wish to read the book once, from cover to cover, to get a general feel for the techniques used, before systematically going over each section. Interview preparation can be quite intense, particularly if you have a long way to go. Brainstorming, structuring and delivering answers can be tiring if you do too much in one go. You should ideally you should take on one section at a time so that you have time to assimilate the information, work on it, and practise and refine your approach.

If you are pressed for time or if your interview is imminent
If you are under pressure, or simply too busy to spend much time preparing, you may wish to read the section on key interview techniques first and then select 10 to 20 key questions to work on before the interview, spanning a range of topics. It is best to spend quality time (i.e. 5–10 minutes per question) preparing a limited number of questions than to prepare hundreds of questions at a rate of 5 seconds each. At the interview, you will have to make two minutes out of your five seconds of preparation, and the result could prove quite painful (e.g. you might either freeze, or start waffling to buy time). Technique and quality are more important than quantity. This modular approach enables you to prepare effectively, whether you have an interview tomorrow, next week or in a few months' time.

Health warning

In this book, we have provided examples of good and bad answers. Their purpose is to give you an appreciation of what sounds good and bad, and how answers can be improved. so that you can apply a similar thinking process to your own answers. There are many types of bad answers, but there are also many types of good answers. The examples in this book should be taken as illustrations of the techniques discussed and not as a blanket template for all your answers. Instead of replicating each answer faithfully, try to use it to understand each of the principles outlined and to determine how you can then apply these principles to your own situation.

Every candidate is unique and it is pretty much impossible to provide examples that are suitable for all candidates in every specialty. Whenever possible, we have explained how the content can be adapted to the various specialties. What is important is that you understand the techniques and mode of thinking behind the answer, so that you can adapt them to your own specialty and circumstances.

THE
SELECTION
PROCESS

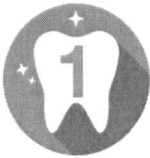

Structure of the interview

Recruitment to dental specialties at ST1 entry point is nationally driven, with single-shot approaches at selection centres. Recruitment for each specialty is often led by a particular region of Health Education England (e.g. in 2019 Health Education England North West organised the ST1 intake for restorative dentistry). Interviews may vary in format between specialties, but most have common themes and structures. All are multiple-station affairs. with multiple assessors at each and multiple marking opportunities.

Before attending your interview, make sure that you know the format adopted for your specialty. as this will influence the way in which you need to respond. You may need to be concise, to work to a specified time frame in your answers. In addition, some specialities may require pre-interview work to be prepared.

Stations can be split between:

- Clinical skills stations (beyond the scope of the current textbook and reliant on your clinical skills and abilities as a safe practitioner, with potential for developing advanced skills, i.e. not yet the finished product)
- Formal interview stations (i.e. traditional question-and-answer sessions)
- Practical interview stations (e.g. involving role players)

In addition, some specialities such as dental core training (DCT) and dental foundation training (DFT) recruitment use situational judgement tests (SJTs). These are reliant on safe practice and "right" decision making, as opposed to breadth and depth of clinical knowledge. Applicants are assessed on:

- Appraisal and decision making
- Coping with pressure
- Critical thinking
- Professionalism
- Patient-centred care

More information can be found on guidance documents for DCT application, published on the East Midlands Deanery website.[1]

---

[1] https://www.eastmidlandsdeanery.nhs.uk/sites/default/files/dct_applicant_guide_2019.pdf

1.1 Formal interview stations

These are reminiscent of the old-style "chat", but don't be fooled. Generally speaking, these interviews feature multiple assessors, scoring you against "anchor statements" within a rigid marking system. There is little room for manoeuvre, and marks that are widely deviated from the mean may be discounted or queried.

Portfolio station

This is your chance to shine and score easy points before even opening your mouth. The introduction of a requirement of a validated logbook sees many candidates start off behind the start line by neglecting to secure validation in advance of the interview day. Portfolios may be marked either whilst you are sitting with the assessors or when you are out of the room, depending upon the level and specialty you are applying to. Here are some key pointers:

- Make your portfolio distinctive but understated. It should stand out, as it is your envoy or ambassador in the interview process. If everyone else has the stock ring binder, whilst you have a crisp, white file with a printed personalised cover, the assessors may arguably be well disposed towards you before even opening the cover.
- Make everything easy to find. Assessors will have a limited amount of time to score your portfolio against strict marking criteria. If they are unable to locate the information they need, they are well within their rights to withhold marks accordingly.
- Lay the portfolio out exactly as specified in the instructions given to you in advance of the interview day. Assessors are notoriously unforgiving towards candidates who deviate from these instructions.
- Be realistic about the volume of information you are presenting. If you have three years of post-graduate experience, you should not be bringing your portfolio in in a wheelbarrow! Assessors like to see a selective display of achievements. It is telling that at most conferences the most junior staff run over time when talking about their minor audit projects, whilst the full-time PhD student is able to keep to time when talking about three years of research. Being concise and to the point is an art.
- Remember, there is only one thing worse than the assessors being unable to find a piece of information in your portfolio. That is you being unable to find it! Know it like the back of your hand, index it well and practise finding relevant items quickly and effortlessly.

Management station (including teamwork, NHS and GDC knowledge)

This question hinges on your understanding of wider issues being faced by the specialty. As sad as it may sound, you are essentially being interviewed for membership into a "club". Interviewers who have given up their time to recruit new trainees can feel quite passionate about their "club" and want to see that you understand the landscape. You may even be asked about NHS hot topics relevant to the specialty in hand (e.g. commissioning for orthognathic surgery in orthodontics; the role of managed clinical networks in oral surgery).

Above and beyond this, specialty training does not aim to just produce proficient clinicians, but also to make trainees leaders and innovators in their field. Assessors are looking for the germs of this idea in prospective candidates.

The focus may also be on multidisciplinary working, interfacing with other specialties, and the interpersonal relationship standards laid out by the GDC to all its registrants.

Clinical experience and commitment to specialty station

In this type of station, you should aim to demonstrate core fundamental skills, to use as building blocks in moving towards competence and then proficiency in higher training. Ideally, assessors want to see evidence of early commitment to the specialty (e.g. membership of the British Orthodontic Society, presentations at regional/national events). You may need to think outside the box in applying lessons learnt in other specialties, but assessors will look favourably upon your ability to cross-pollinate ideas from other specialties. For example, dental specialties interface heavily with each other, and it is no bad thing for a prospective orthodontic trainee to have an understanding and experience of paediatric dentistry.

Clinical governance station

Questions may resolve around the following:

- Your practical understanding of clinical governance and how it affects your clinical practice (e.g. "What do you understand by clinical governance?", "How does clinical governance impact upon your daily practice?").
- Evidence-based dentistry (EBD) and guidelines (e.g. "How do you deliver EBD to your patients?", "Tell me about a recent article that changed your clinical practice", or "Tell me about a recent guideline that has influenced the delivery of care in this specialty.").
- Risk management (e.g. "Tell me about a recent mistake you have made", "What is a root cause analysis?", "What is a never event?", or "What happens to Datix® forms once submitted?").

Academic/research station

This station may exist as a standalone station (particularly in recruitment to academic clinical fellow (ACF) posts) or be encompassed elsewhere. Essentially, the aim is to test your understanding and experience of teaching, research and audit. These are all integral skills to any future clinical leader in the NHS, but particularly true of future academics. Questions may be:

- Factual, e.g. "How do you critically appraise a paper?" or "Tell me about your experience of the audit process"
- Reflective, e.g. "What did you gain from your research experience?" or "Tell me about a bad experience you had in delivering teaching"
- Contentious, e.g. "Do you think that all trainees should be involved in research?"

If you are applying for an ACF post, you should ideally have a broad idea of the research areas that interest you, how they align with prospective supervisors, and how you might lay the groundwork and secure funding for a higher degree (DDS/PhD) in later years. You should also demonstrate a good understanding of the academic career pathway, exit points and plans to ensure career progression.

Clinical scenario station

This will test your ability to handle difficult workplace-based problems that may hinge on stretching your abilities, contentious areas of practice, interprofessional working, unrealistic patient expectations/complaints, ethical dilemmas, and many other variations, which we will explore more in this book. Past interviews have included the following:

- Managing two or more important matters at the same time, e.g. the carer/parent of a patient with special needs who passes out during an extraction, effectively creating two patients
- Approaching a task for which you are not fully qualified, e.g. an unforeseen surgical complication that you have not previously encountered, such as a displaced third molar root into the sublingual space
- Dealing with substandard/unethical treatment and/or a lack of integrity, e.g. a dental nurse who fails to sterilise impressions before sending them off, a drunken colleague, or a junior trainee who is always late

1.2 **Practical interview stations**

Practical stations involve more hands-on work. They feature nearly all specialties. Rather than testing your knowledge base, they are assessing your ability to demonstrate good interpersonal skills, mature and sound judgement, and decision making commensurate with the level of training and the potential for further development in higher training.

Clinical communication station

This is essentially a "role play" or "simulated patient consultation" station. You are given a small amount of time (usually 5–10 minutes) to engage with an actor playing the part of a patient. Generally, there are common themes, e.g. a complaint, an unmet expectation (which may or may not be realistic), or breaking bad news. Communication stations help assessors examine your interpersonal skills rather than your specialty knowledge, and it is easy to forget this. Assessors may actually deduct marks for overuse of jargon, unclear and cumbersome explanations, and a failure to develop a rapport. It is all about pitching your explanations/apologies to the level of the patient and meeting their expectations.

Objective structured clinical examination (OSCE)-style assessments

These may be substituted by clinical skills assessments in most specialties, but they featured as a separate component in oral surgery recruitment in 2019 by HEE Yorkshire and the Humber. There were five separate, structured assessments, one lasting 20 minutes and the others lasting 20 minutes. OSCEs may hinge on demonstration of data interpretation, examination findings and interpretation of radiographs or histology reports. If you are competent to an appropriate level in your job and can think laterally, then you should have no problem in demonstrating your skills in a viva situation and in answering any clinical questions thrown at you. Doubts in this regard may be better addressed using appropriate clinical textbooks and revision materials, as well as optimising clinical time in the run-up to the interview, by seeing more challenging patients under consultant supervision, or through via discussion of strengths and weaknesses with educational super visors and other senior colleagues.

Presentation stations

Presentations more commonly feature in consultant interviews these days but can still make an appearance in some specialty recruitment. Candidates may be given the topic ahead of schedule or on the day, with minimal resources (e.g. a flipchart). We dedicate a separate chapter to these stations in case you encounter them, but the key point is to be concise but comprehensive. Slides should not be overly text-heavy, and you should be talking around them rather than reading them if using a presentation software such as Microsoft PowerPoint. Nobel prize-winning physicist Richard Feynman once said that if you can't explain something in simple terms, you probably don't fully understand it yourself. Themes may be:

- Generic, e.g. why you want to do this specialty
- Political, e.g. the future of orthognathic surgery in the commissioning era
- Personal, e.g. what interests you outside of dentistry

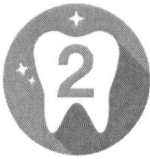

2 Selection criteria

Most interviews in dentistry are "structured". They are aiming, in a methodical approach, to identify key skills, attributes and qualities that meet the criteria for a successful applicant who is going to be good at the job. This is distinct from the "unstructured" approach in years past of an informal "chat" with candidates. Interviewers are tasked with establishing:

- Competence to perform the job
- A demonstration of the right attitude
- Whether or not the applicant will "fit in"

A portion of the assessment in these domains happens before you set foot in the interview, through the scoring of your application form and/or your CV. You should ensure you are familiar with the person specification for the job and that you meet the essential (and preferably all/most of the desirable) criteria. This holds true for your approach in filling in the application form and in tailoring your response to questions asked at interview. This is not a "one size fits all" approach and is very much a case of being right for the job on offer. Your application and interview should reflect your understanding of the criteria being tested.

To understand what is required, you should look at:

- The national person specification for the specialty you are applying to, many of which can be found on the COPDEND website[2]
- The General Dental Council (GDC) document *Standards for the Dental Team*[3]

---

[2] https://www.copdend.org/postgraduate-training/national-person-specification/
[3] https://standards.gdc-uk.org/Assets/pdf/Standards%20for%20the%20Dental%20Team.pdf

2.1   National person specification

The national person specification for each specialty lays out clearly and concisely what is expected of candidates. Specifications are usually divided into essential and desirable criteria, the former making you eligible for selection and the latter making you the preferred candidate. It is unlikely that you will comprehensively comply with all of the desirable criteria, and you are likely to have areas of strength that differ from those of your competitors. The important thing is to know the national person specification for your specialty inside out so that you know what they are looking for in a future trainee. This will enable you to shape your answers to match the anchor statements with the most marks and pitch yourself right at interview.

National person specifications can be found for each of the dental specialties on the lead deanery website for that specialty, e.g. Health Education England North East was lead deanery for orthodontics in 2019. National person specifications are quite formulaic and follow a similar pattern, as outlined below.

Qualifications

By the time you get to the interview stage, there is little you can do about your qualifications. Make sure your application form reflects accurately the qualifications that you have gained, though. Generally speaking, the essential criterion is a BDS/BChD or equivalent, recognised by the General Dental Council. Additional points are gained for membership diplomas such as the MFDS/MJDF, and higher degrees such as MSc/DDS/PhD, or even intercalated qualifications, e.g. BSc.

Career progression

Again, at interview stage, your career progression is set. Evidence of foundation competencies and dental core training year 2 completion at the point of entry is mandatory for specialty recruitment (ST1). Desirable criteria include: being on a performers' list or able to meet requirements for listing, evidence of attending courses commensurate with the level of training, and having experience from more than one dental specialty/clinical setting.

Clinical skills

Essential criteria include:

- Good patient care skills
- Capacity to apply sound judgement to clinical problems
- Ability to prioritise clinical need

- Appropriate technical and clinical competence
- Development of diagnostic skills and clinical judgement commensurate with training level/experience

At the interview, these may be tested by asking you:

- To describe a difficult case that you have managed
- To describe a difficult situation where you had to prioritise clinical needs
- To explain how you would resolve a specific clinical situation
- To prioritise clinical needs in a simulated scenario
- To analyse test results and/or images and describe the next most logical step in the management process
- To demonstrate a given practical skill
- To demonstrate your understanding of risk management

Problem solving and decision making feature heavily here. They rely on the ability to be logical and exhibit lateral thinking, to solve problems and make decisions. You should be able to think beyond the obvious and be flexible in your approach, demonstrating the capacity to bring a range of approaches to problem solving. Problem-solving skills are often best examined by confronting candidates with clinical dilemmas or difficult scenarios, where there are no "easy" or "right" answers. Questions that may probe these areas specifically include being asked:

- To discuss a situation where you had to make a difficult decision (e.g. without senior support)
- To handle a simulated scenario (e.g. more junior colleague inadvertently extracting the wrong tooth)
- To give an example of a scenario where you showed initiative
- To describe how you would deal with a difficult clinical situation

Academic/research skills

Essential criteria include:

- Understanding of the principles and relevance of research in evidence-based practice
- Understanding of the principles of audit / clinical governance / quality improvement
- Evidence of participation in quality improvement / audit / service evaluation

Desirable criteria include:

- Relevant academic and research achievements, e.g. awards

- Publications
- Conference presentations/posters
- Leading a quality improvement project
- Evidence of delivering undergraduate/postgraduate teaching
- Teaching qualifications, e.g. PGCert Med Ed or similar

At the interview, these may be tested by asking you:

- To discuss the importance of your research and audit experience
- To explain the difference between audit and research
- To demonstrate your understanding of the audit cycle
- To discuss the usefulness of audit in clinical practice
- To debate the role of research in medical training
- To summarise and analyse a paper that you have read recently
- To explain the principles underlying evidence-based dentistry
- To explain research governance or statistical concepts
- To summarise the extent of your teaching experience
- To debate the efficacy of various teaching methods

Personal skills

Essential criteria include:

- Capacity to communicate effectively and sensitively with others
- Ability to discuss treatment/oral health options with patients/stakeholders in a way they can understand
- Ability to demonstrate good information technology skills
- Capacity to think beyond the obvious, with analytical and flexible mind, bringing a range of approaches to problem solving
- Ability to demonstrate effective judgement and decision-making skills
- Capacity to work effectively in a multidisciplinary team
- Capacity to establish good working relationships with others

The remit of personal skills in the national person specifications often encompasses managing others, leadership and team playing, as well as organisation and planning (e.g. prioritising tasks, following instructions) and vigilance and situational awareness (e.g. anticipating and adapting to situations that may change rapidly). Candidates are also examined for the ability to cope with pressure and manage uncertainty, awareness of their own limitations and willingness to ask for help, decisiveness and resilience.

With regard to judgement and coping with pressure, this may be tested by asking you:

- How you handle stress
- To provide an example of a situation where you were stressed
- To explain how you would handle a given stressful scenario
- To give an example of a mistake you made
- To talk about a recent situation in which you had to ask for senior help or where you felt out of your depth
- To describe a situation where you had to make decisions in a changing environment
- To ask about your weaknesses
- To discuss how you deal with criticism

Managing others may be examined by asking you:

- To explain what makes you a good team player or leader
- To provide examples of when you have played an important role in a team or demonstrated good leadership
- To detail your experience of working in teams
- To explain what makes a good team and to discuss the advantages and disadvantages of working in teams
- To provide an example of a time when you had to deal with a difficult situation at work
- To detail your experience of managing others
- To discuss the difference between management and leadership
- To discuss how you delegate and/or to provide examples of delegation and management

Organisation and planning may be assessed by asking you:

- To explain how you manage your workload or your time
- To provide an example of a situation where you had to prioritise
- To prioritise a list of five of six emergencies or other tasks
- To explain how you would organise a ward round, a theatre list or a training session
- To detail your IT experience and explain its relevance

Vigilance and situational awareness may be tested by asking you:

- To provide an example where your showed initiative
- To provide an example of a time when you had to remain vigilant
- To describe a situation when you resolved an unsafe situation

- To explain how you ensure that you remain fully aware of what is happening in complex clinical situations
- To discuss how you would handle a given clinical scenario, e.g. a collapse in the clinic

Probity / professional integrity

Probity is assessed in line with GDC guidance outlined below, but anchor statements regard the following as essential criteria:

- Taking responsibility for actions
- Demonstrating honesty and reliability
- Demonstrating respect for the rights of all
- Demonstrating awareness of ethical principles, safety, confidentiality and consent
- Demonstrating awareness of the importance of being the patient's advocate, clinical governance, and the responsibilities of an NHS employee

The demonstration of altruism is regarded as desirable and was described, in the generic portion of the person specification for the dental specialties in 2019, as "evidence of the ability to attend to the needs of others with an awareness of their rights and equal opportunities".

Specialty-specific criteria

Specialty-specific criteria are above and beyond the generic requirements and, as the term implies, these vary between dental specialties. Validated logbooks, experience of working within the dental specialty in question, realistic insight into the career and a demonstration of commitment to the specialty are generally required. Desirable criteria may include:

- Experience in allied specialties
- Attendance at / participation in national/international meetings
- Publication and/or presentation
- Awareness of the training programme pathway
- Participation in courses, e.g. IV sedation, ILS
- Membership of appropriate societies, e.g. British Orthodontic Society (BOS)

2.2 GDC guidance

The GDC's *Standards for the Dental Team* and other documents

The guidance available through the GDC talks about the responsibilities and behaviours expected of dental professionals, with respect to colleagues and the public. Standards and guidance are available online[4] and include:

1. Standards for the dental team
2. GDC guidance for dental professionals
3. Principles for handling complaints
4. Direct access
5. Scope of practice

Spend some time becoming familiar with these documents and their contents. You will not be quizzed directly on them, but you will need to use them to construct and shape your answers in areas such as professional dilemma questions. They should be used as your "touchstone" to inform your answer, as anchoring statements in mark sheets are likely to be based on their contents as an objective standard.

In particular, the GDC focuses on nine principles:

1. Put patients' interests first
2. Communicate effectively with patients
3. Obtain valid consent
4. Maintain and protect patients' information
5. Have a clear and effective complaints procedure
6. Work with colleagues in a way that is in the patients' best interests
7. Maintain, develop and work within your professional knowledge and skills
8. Raise concerns if patients are at risk
9. Make sure your personal behaviour maintains patients' confidence in you and the dental profession

[4]https://www.gdc-uk.org/information-standards-guidance/standards-and-guidance

FORMAL INTERVIEW STATIONS

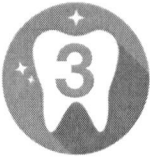

③ Marking scheme

DCT and ST interviews are structured. Questions are designed to assess specific attributes or skills, often in combination, and candidates are marked against a rigid set of criteria.

These are often divided into domains with subthemes, and may be scored against "anchor statements", which give a descriptor of a candidate scoring a particular outcome. For example, a top-scoring candidate may demonstrate attributes such as fluidity of thought, independent decision making, and knowledge above and beyond the expected for their year of training.

The concept of scoring against rigid criteria is done in the interest of fairness and transparency, preventing interviewers from pursuing their own agenda and/or personal interests. That said, there is still a degree of subjectivity on the part of the examiner, with "doves and hawks" still being apparent in the extremes of marking.

Candidates may assume that there is a "right" answer. In theory there Is; however, it is not a verbatim answer but rather an answer that demonstrates maturity, higher-order thinking, the ability to work from basic principles and information and, above all, a safe approach to tackling problems. Interviewers are viewing you as potential future colleagues and, as such, will be expecting you to behave as though you already were.

Positive and negative indicators

For each question, the anchoring statements may be either descriptors of the ideal candidate or a set of positive and negative indicators to score against. They may be labelled this way, or as "competent", "not competent", etc. The theme is universal; the semantics are different.

So, for example, in response to the question "One of your colleagues is underperforming; what would you do?", the indicators might look like this:

Positive indicators	Negative indicators
• Considers impact on patient safety • Considers the impact on the team and colleagues • Remains open-minded • Does not judge or jump to conclusions • Involves appropriate support from / reports appropriately to senior colleagues • Adopts a supportive and constructive approach	• Does not consider the impact on patient safety or on the team • Compromises patient safety • Handles problems alone • Focuses on reporting without measuring the implications on the colleague • Does not involve appropriate team members • Judgemental and unsupportive

For the question "Describe a time when you demonstrated leadership", positive and negative indicators may be as follows:

Positive indicators	Negative indicators
• Adopts an empowering approach and clearly defines roles of others • Acts to unify objectives of the group and utilises skills of others to best advantage • Clearly communicates with the group • Establishes roles and requirements of a team • Works to achieve a good outcome for patients • Flexible leadership style, as appropriate, to emerging challenges in situation	• Overbearing attitude • Singular leadership style • Autocratic approach to leadership • Does not recognise contribution of the team members • Fails to empower others • Poor communication • Unwillingness to relinquish control when appropriate • Not concerned with overall outcome / patient safety

There may be prompting from interviewers if you fail to hit key considerations but they feel you are on the right track. However, prompting tends to lead to a deduction in marks.

Positive and negative indicators are generally imposed by central recruitment offices or the lead region. All candidates will therefore be judged according to the same indicators within the same specialty recruitment. Arguably, in the pursuit of generic skills and raw potential rather than the finished product, there are generic competencies and skills in positive and negative predictors, which lend themselves to ANY specialty recruitment.

Marking schedule

Based on the indicators, interviewers will be charged with scoring on a scale. This may be done globally for the question as a whole and/or within separate domains, e.g. "clinical knowledge", "developing dentist–patient rapport". Scores may be numerical on a continuum (e.g. out of 10, out of 20), ordinal using numbers (e.g. 0–5, with 5 being the "best" anchor statement and 0 being the "worst"), or ordinal using words (e.g. bad, poor, borderline fail, borderline pass, good, excellent).

One example is provided below as a guide. This is taken from the ST1 clinical governance scenario station descriptors for 2019 specialty training recruitment to orthodontics, freely available online at the time of writing.[5]

0	**Very Poor**	• Unable to answer the question • Largely incomplete and poorly constructed answer • Seriously incorrect, irrelevant, with lack of argument or incoherent contribution • No evidence of basic reading • Presentation untidy with little evidence of knowledge or understanding
1	**Poor**	• Made some attempt to answer the question but not adequate • Failure to develop one or more major strands inherent in the questions • A tendency to irrelevance and failure to argue cogently • Needs to demonstrate more understanding, fewer errors and/or a more willing contribution • Presentation disorganised

[5]https://madeinheene.hee.nhs.uk/Portals/13/Clinical%20Governance%20Station%202019%20-%20Descriptors.pdf

2	**Acceptable**	• A structured answer with essential element correct and no deficiency in basic knowledge and understanding
3	**Good**	• A good clear and willing contribution with minor omissions • Demonstrates understanding of the subject with evidence of further reading • Analysis rather than description of relevant detail
4	**Outstanding**	• Represents the best that can be expected at this stage of the candidate's career • Completely correct and literate showing a thorough knowledge and understanding of the subject area, a high degree of relevance and referenced when appropriate

In a few marking schemes, some negative indicators may be "decisive", i.e. they will automatically push you towards a lower grade, by virtue of being more heavily weighted due to the seriousness of the issues they represent. In the main, these relate to patient safety. Whilst it may be "forgivable" to omit to talk about having a flexible style of leadership, failing to report a colleague who is putting patients at risk could score you an automatic 0 or, at the very least, pull you down the scoreboard considerably. Many interview score sheets feature a "red box" to highlight probity concerns, when there is cause for concern relating to behaviour fundamentally contradicting the guidance of the GDC.

Throughout this book, we will look at anchor statements, scoring systems and positive and negative indicators for a wide range of questions. This will give you an idea of how to pitch your answers and what to aim for. It will also enable you to work from basic principles when addressing unexpected questions, and "second-guess" what interviewers are really looking for in a candidate.

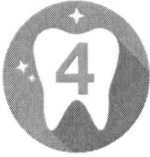

4 Key interview techniques

The following techniques will help you ensure that your answers come across as convincing, meaningful and confident.

Keep your answers concise – maximum 2 minutes

No one can listen to a speaker for in excess of 1.5 to 2 minutes, unless the subject matter is inherently fascinating and/or there are accompanying audio-visual aids. Your interviewers will be seeing in excess of 30 candidates per day and you must ensure they remain alert. They will therefore be looking for answers that "get to the point".

Conversely, having answers that are too short may give the impression that you are not investing any effort in the process, so 1.5 to 2 minutes is about right. You can make an exception in response to open-ended questions such as "Tell me about your training to date" or "Take me through your CV", which require you to provide a lot more information than a standard question would. However, even with these, three minutes is the maximum amount of time that you should spend on your answer.

In dental specialty interviews, some stations may feature four or five structured questions as a scenario evolves. In the context of a 10-minute station, offering 1.5- to 2-minute answers will allow breathing space for the interviewers to ask the questions and expand on any points that require further clarification.

Avoid long introductions – answer the questions directly

The interviewers are interested in you – they want your personal take on the answer. Being asked "What is your experience of clinical governance?" does not mean that they wish you to define clinical governance. Imagine listening to 36 candidates in sequence, all defining clinical governance. Aside from the fact it would be very boring, nobody wants a trainee who regurgitates a Wikipedia entry!

Many candidates would start the answer to the clinical governance question with "Clinical governance consists of 7 pillars, …". The question is not asking you to name the 7 pillars; so, spending time listing them would eat into the two-minute window far too much. An outstanding candidate would provide three or four meaningful examples of their own involvement in clinical governance, which not only showcase their understanding of the concept, but also some of their achievements to date.

Similarly, when asked "Describe your communication skills", telling the interviewer how important communication skills are for your specialty of choice misses the point. Rather, an excellent answer would go something along the lines of: "I feel that I have good communication skills and have received feedback in the form of 360-degree appraisals and multi-source feedback from patients and colleagues attesting to this. I am clear and concise in both my written and verbal communication, using a structured approach and gauging the needs and understanding of the recipient of any information I am imparting. For instance, in my approach to younger patients, I will always endeavour to explain things in non-threatening and easily understandable ways, whilst simultaneously addressing any concerns their parents might have. I will often conclude consultations by checking understanding, providing written information leaflets (many of which I have helped formulate myself) and directing my letters to parents, to reinforce the messages imparted, copying in the general dental practitioners for their information ...."

The candidate is being asked to describe their own communication skills and not to discuss the generic importance of communication skills. Addressing the question generically only serves to irritate interviewers, who are left sitting there under a constrained interviewing system, thinking "This is not addressing the question I asked!"

As a rule, it is sensible to avoid abbreviations or acronyms, even familiar ones. From a communication point of view, they sound sloppy and lazy. You also risk confusing members of the panel if these are regional/local habits rather than specialty-specific ones and/or if you have lay people on your panel.

Demonstrate a shared language

Remember that people are looking for a member of their "club" in allowing you access into their dental specialty. Whilst abbreviations are to be avoided, easily comprehensible, shared terminologies that give a glimpse of your insight and understanding of common bonds (and threats) within the specialty are valuable. Talking about tiers of oral surgery commissioning, for instance, and the allocation of these between different types of oral surgery providers, relies on you understanding the landscape but also being able to "talk the talk". Reading around the subject in advance of the interview and talking about these issues with senior clinicians within your current department may go a long way to "immersing" you in the culture and terminology, without needing to resort to obfuscation.

Structure your answer in three of four points

It is easy to get "lost" in answers and lose your thread. Rather than learning answers verbatim, having a structure is valuable in making the answer clear and serving as a mnemonic. Keep to three or four points as a maximum. So, for example, "Tell me about your teaching experience" could be addressed with the following points:

- Who you taught, in what capacity and where
- What teaching methods you employed
- What formal training you have had in teaching
- What feedback you received and how this has shaped your teaching

Similarly, for "Tell me about a mistake you have made":

- The circumstances surrounding the mistake
- How you dealt with the mistake
- The resolution and outcome
- Your reflective learning on the mistake

Similarly, more open-ended questions should be restricted to three or four mini-examples, with expansion within those subheadings. As an example, consider the question, "What are your main strengths?" You might answer:

- Dynamic and proactive
- Approachable and supportive
- Self-starter and constantly willing to learn and develop

The points can be developed further and expanded upon with examples of practice, to enable interviewers to latch on to your answer and follow an overarching structure.

Expand on each point and illustrate with examples

It is all too easy to quote a few buzzwords, thinking that they will be sufficient to tick the right boxes. For example, many candidates might answer the question "What qualities do you think would make you a good orthodontist?" with the following one-liner: "I feel I would excel in orthodontics because I am hardworking, motivated, dedicated, enthusiastic, and a good team player and communicator." This is essentially a series of generic buzzwords, which, whilst not "wrong", does not convey anything about the candidate individually. It is a very impersonal answer, which risks sounding clichéd and not thought through.

Making broad statements makes you sound vague (and potentially arrogant) and fails to differentiate you from other candidates. After listening to 30 candidates in succession, people sit up and take note of a "fresh" candidate who is delivering a personal answer, peppered with lived experience.

For example, "I learn from experience and constantly seek to develop new skills" is an easy statement to make but could be embellished with personal experience:

> "From the very start of my training, I have taken every opportunity to learn from experiences and opportunities available. In my paediatric dentistry block I learnt a lot of transferable techniques in terms of managing anxious patients, and the use of adjuncts such as inhalational sedation. I recognised a need to hone my skills in this area and attended postgraduate courses, receiving certification from the Society for Advancement of Anaesthesia in Dentistry. I have also conducted an audit of sedation method selection, which was presented at a national meeting and further deepened my understanding of anxious patient management ...."

You can see that the answer above demonstrates:

1. Reflective learning in response to self-identified learning needs, characteristic of a good adult learner
2. Breadth of areas, including governance, clinical acumen and continuing professional development
3. A transferable attitude towards challenges and opportunities, which is likely to "follow" the trainee into their postgraduate training

Ultimately, the answer sounds more mature, individual and natural than the one-liner above.

Signpost each point clearly

Signposting means stating clearly the new concept or idea that you are addressing. Many candidates have answers that are well structured and contain a lot of interesting information, backed up with good examples; however, in spite of this, it can still be difficult to extract the message or idea they are trying to communicate from their answer. This section aims to help you to clarify your message. Once you have a structure in mind, make sure your key messages are announced clearly within each section of your answer. These may be introduced in several ways, as illustrated below.

- **Signposting at the start**
  Signposting is most easily done at the start of each section. For example, an answer to the question "Why do you want to train in orthodontics?" could consist of three sections, signposted as follows:

Introduction	"There are many reasons why I am keen to train in orthodontics.
Signpost and expand	"First, I draw a lot of personal satisfaction from building a personal rapport with patients and looking after them over a long treatment course, helping them to see it through <expand why and how, with examples>.
Signpost and expand	"As well as this, I also have a strong interest in research and feel that orthodontics is an excellent specialty in which to pursue that interest. <expand, explaining what your research interests might be and how you would follow these in higher training and beyond>
Signpost and expand	"Finally, I really enjoy working as part of a multidisciplinary team, achieving the best outcomes for patients with complex treatment needs, where many heads are better than one. <expand on how this is important in orthodontics and what you enjoy about it and derive from it>"

In this sample, each section starts with a clear message, which is what the candidate wants the interviewers to remember about him/her.

- **Signposting at the end**

  In this instance, the candidate describes experience at the outset and then summarises each point with a description of how this is relevant to the question being asked. For instance, if asked the question "Why do you want to train in dental public health?", instead of stating up front that he/she has a strong interest in research, the candidate could phrase the answer as follows:

Context/experience	"During my dental core training period, I had the opportunity to become involved in two research projects, one on <xxx>, and another one on <yyy>. Through my involvement in these projects, I gained a good insight into different research methodologies and the importance of research overall. I helped secure funding, contributed to the application for ethics approval,

	collected data and helped with the analysis and write-up. I felt very at ease with clinical and academic components of the job.
Signpost	"I feel that dental public health will help me build on this initial foundation in research, allowing me to apply these research skills to improve population dental health."

There would then be more sections dealing with other reasons for choosing dental public health as a career. Each time, the summary sentence clearly states the message raised and leaves the interviewers with no ambiguity as to what the candidate is trying to say.

- **Vary the signposting**
  Beginning all sections of all answers with a signpost is likely to make you sound slightly "military" or overly systematic. Signposting all sections at the end may give the feeling that you are constantly trying to build suspense and drama in your answers.

  If you can, i.e. if you feel confident enough to do so, try to vary the ways in which you signpost so that some of your answers have points that are signposted at the start and others at the end. This will give a more balanced picture and will be easier on the ear of your panel.

  However, if you do not feel able to vary your answers in this way, stick to signposting at the start. It is the easier of the two to master. Once you feel more comfortable, you can start experimenting and softening your delivery, by mixing the two styles.

Use power words and active verbs

Selling yourself is not just about stating your message clearly and describing your experience. It is also about sounding confident, mature and, generally speaking, in control. It is a common mistake for candidates to understate their experience. In order to appear more confident, you will need to adopt a vocabulary that may be slightly different from that which you are accustomed to on a day-to-day basis, and which will sell you in an active and enthusiastic manner.

There is no need to learn a whole list of words in order to achieve this. When you are preparing your answers to some of the more common questions, particularly those based on your personal experience, you should question whether your answers sound energetic and enthusiastic enough. If they don't, this could be a problem with the structure or a lack of personalisation in your answer; but it could also be due to the lack of power words and active verbs.

Example

"After a few attempts, I was able to reach a compromise with my colleagues, as I am quite good at interprofessional working"

On the surface, it sounds like a good thing to say. However, "After a few attempts" and "I was able to" sound weak. They make it sound as if the candidate didn't try that hard or is not particularly proud of their achievement. The sentence could have a much stronger impact if it were reworded as follows:

Revised statement

"My training to date has made me comfortable and proficient at seeing the viewpoints of others in situations that would benefit from cross-specialty working. In this instance, I was able to recognise and clarify the viewpoints of other clinicians involved, but succeeded in achieving a compromise that translated to the best possible care and outcome for the patient."

In addition to the power words and enthusiasm, there is clear ownership of the situation, something we will come onto further in the next section.

Talk about yourself, and not everyone else

Candidates often make the mistake of talking about everything and everyone else, other than themselves. Dentistry and the dental specialties are "team sports", and there is a temptation to talk repeatedly about "we" and "the team". Whilst this does present a good team-player attitude and ethic, it detracts from the opportunity to sell individual skills and competencies.

In your interview, it is perfectly acceptable to introduce some collective actions and make statements such as "As a team, we were charged with conducting an audit on the quality of radiographs taken within the practice". This sentence should, however, serve as an introduction to the rest of the answer, which remains focused on you and your individual contribution, e.g. "My responsibilities were ...".

Remember that they are not interviewing the team and not offering the team a job. At the back of many interviewers' minds is the thought that you may have been "coasting". We all know people who can put a line on their CV to say "they did" a particular job in a particular department, but this can mean very different things to different individuals. Explain what you gained from situations and opportunities, what your contributions were and what lessons you learned.

Bring objectivity into your answers

If you feel awkward talking about yourself or don't want to appear boastful, a good way to overcome this problem is to bring objectivity into your answers. This can be achieved by:

1. Illustrating your answers with personal examples
2. Mentioning feedback that you have received, either informally or through 360-degree appraisal

Instead of saying "I feel that I am a caring dentist", you may feel more comfortable saying that "Patients and colleagues alike have often commented that I go the extra mile in providing care and that I am meticulous in ascertaining patient need and expectations and tailoring my treatment plans accordingly".

Avoid making vague statements, being definite and factual instead. Avoid saying things like "I went into orthodontics because I like it", but rather back the statement up. Say why you like about it (e.g. the ability to be involved with patients over sustained time periods, the confidence that you see your patients develop throughout treatment), give concrete examples that highlight your skills (e.g. the satisfaction questionnaires that you asked your patients to complete at the end of treatment) and, above all, say why you are suited to it (e.g. your patience, your attention to detail). Use facts to substantiate your general statements.

Avoid unnecessary detail

Avoid excessive detail unless you have been asked for specifics. If you provide too much detail, you risk making your answers very lengthy and wordy. Most importantly, you will distract from your key messages by concentrating on one issue, whilst the question may be looking for a much broader response.

Remain positive

It is astonishing how many candidates will undersell themselves with negative statements such as, "Well, I haven't done much research", or "I am reasonably competent at <xxx>." To make an impact, you must sell what you have rather than what you don't have. It is a natural tendency of altruistic, self-sacrificing healthcare professionals to shy away from self-promotion. For the purposes of an interview, however, this attitude needs to be parked. There is no need to be arrogant; but saying what you can do and, moreover, what you are proficient in, with a positive attitude, will go a long way.

If you don't show that you believe in yourself, then no one else will.

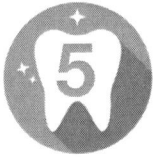

5 Key interview structures and frameworks

In order to produce structured and meaningful answers, you will need to learn to use a number of structures and frameworks, which will make your life easier. Once you have mastered these, you will be able to apply them endlessly across a wide range of questions. Not only will this give you a sense of direction, it will also provide you with reassurance as you deliver your answers. You will feel more in control because you will know that there are sound principles that you can apply, regardless of what the question is.

In this section, we introduce three fundamental structures:

- **CAMP** – for background and motivation questions
- **STAR** – for skills-based questions asking for specific examples
- **SPIES** – to answer questions on difficult colleagues or conflicts

Make sure that you do not simply memorise these techniques but that you learn to use them intelligently – the next level beyond the use of acronyms to simply remember, for example, the cranial nerves or branches of the internal iliac artery. At the interview, you are likely to feel nervous and to blank out if you simply try to recall information. The key to success is to allow sufficient time to prepare, so that these structures become second nature and you do not have to do so much thinking and information-recalling on the spot.

Throughout the book, we will apply these key generic structures and will also develop other structures that are more specific to individual questions. More importantly, we will show you how to think about the questions logically and construct answers, using your common sense and experience.

5.1 The CAMP structure (for background and motivation questions)

CAMP = Clinical, Academic, Management, Personal

When answering questions such as "Tell me about yourself" or "Tell me about your training to date", or being asked to work through your portfolio, CAMP will provide you with a ready-made structure, which will enable you to provide a logical and well-developed answer. For example, when asked "Tell me why you wish to consider a career in oral medicine", CAMP may prompt you to approach the answer as follows:

Clinical	You may talk about jobs you have had to date that provide a foundation in key skills relevant to the role (e.g. DCT level work in oral medicine). You may also talk about complementary specialty experience (e.g. time spend in maxillofacial surgery as a DCT), or about courses you have attended and objective evidence of achievements (e.g. work-based assessments such as CbDs in an oral medicine clinic).
Academic	You may talk about research work you have been involved in that is relevant to oral medicine. This may have led to a higher qualification or intercalated degree, and you may have plans for a DDS/PhD in your higher training, allowing you to talk about this. You may have presented groundwork in this area nationally or internationally. You may have a teaching qualification (e.g. PGCert) and express a wish to contribute to the undergraduate teaching.
Management	You may have been involved in QI projects to date that have equipped you with a transferable skillset and/or project idea to cross-pollinate service development between units. Maybe you have been the trainee rep at a junior level, or have designs on setting up a study club or regional BDA meeting.
Personal	You may have interests that demonstrate an ingrained personal attitude to bettering yourself and achieving. This need not be an Olympic medal, but simply progressing from a 5K park run to a half marathon. You may have interests that chime with other people in the department, that are unique/unusual, or that simply mean you are likely to be happy in a particular place.

5.2 The STAR structure
(for questions asking for an example)

STAR = Situation, Task, Action, Result/Reflect

This method of structuring answers lends itself particularly well to questions asking for specific examples such as:

- "Tell us about a situation where you worked under pressure."
- "Describe a situation when you dealt with a difficult patient."
- "Tell us about a time when you played a key role in a team."
- "Describe a situation where you had to ask for senior help."
- "Give an example where your communication skills made a difference to the care of a patient."

Many interviewers will have been trained to use this structure. Even if they have not, they will recognise its value when they see it. The information will be given to them in a structured manner and, as a result, they will become more receptive to the messages you are trying to communicate.

Interviewers will be looking for the following:

Situation	What is the context of the story?
Task	What did you have to achieve?
Action	What did you do? How did you go about achieving it? And why did you do it in that way?
Result/ **R**eflect	What happened at the end? Why did you feel you did well? What did you learn? How did it change you?

Situation and Task

Describe the situation that you were confronted with and/or the task that needed to be accomplished. This section is merely setting the scene for the "Action" section so that your panel can understand the story from start to finish. You should therefore aim to make it concise and informative, concentrating solely on what is pertinent to the story and the message you are trying to communicate.

For example, if the question is asking you to describe a situation where you had to deal with a difficult person, explain how you came to meet that person and why they were being difficult. If the question is asking for an example of teamwork, explain the task that you had to undertake as a team and what your role was.

Action

This is the most important section, as it is where you will need to demonstrate that you have the skills and personal attributes that the question is testing. Having set the context of your story, you need to explain the action you took, bearing in mind the following:

- Be personal, i.e. talk about you, not other people.
- Go into some detail. Do not assume that the interviewers will guess what you mean.
- Steer clear of clinical information, unless it is essential for the general comprehension of the story.
- Explain not just what you did, but how and why you did it.

Explain the actions that you took to resolve the situation, clearly highlighting your role. In describing your role, keep in mind the purpose of the question and the skills that it is asking you to demonstrate.

For example, a question asking you to provide an example of a situation when you dealt with a difficult patient will involve discussing a number of points, including:

- How you used your communication skills effectively
- How you sought to involve others in helping you deal with the patient
- How you dealt with your frustration

If you stick to explaining what you did and how you did it, you run the risk of giving an answer that is slightly too basic. In your answer, you must be able to demonstrate that you are taking actions because you understand their purpose and what they will achieve, not simply because you got lucky.

Never lose sight of the fact that the example that you give is of interest only if you demonstrate through your narration how you match the desired criteria.

Consider the following question and (ineffective) answer:

Question

"Tell me about a time where you dealt with a difficult patient encounter."

Ineffective answer

"During my time in oral surgery as a DCT, I was assigned to a general anaesthetic day-surgery list. Part of my duties was consenting patients prior to surgery. I saw one patient who seemed unsure as to whether she was having her ectopic canine tooth exposed or removed. Thankfully, I was able to clarify the plan with the referring dentist and the situation was easily resolved."

The answer is very superficial and, whilst it does follow the STAR structure, there is little in the way of personal involvement, a distinct lack of detail, no evidence of reflection and personal or institutional learning, and overall it is lacking in lustre. We gain no insights as to why the candidate is acting in a particular way and there is a real need to highlight the thinking behind the actions here:

Reworded partial answer

"In this situation, there were a number of issues that I needed to address. First, it was clear that the patient did not actually understand the procedure that was being carried out. In addition, there was conflicting information from different sources, such that it was prudent to seek reassurance from the referring clinician with regard to the definitive treatment plan. Having contacted the orthodontist, I was able to clarify the intended treatment plan and then use this to discuss the operation with the patient, to check their understanding and willingness to proceed."

Explaining actions and the reasoning behind these actions brings more depth to the answers and ultimately results in a higher-scoring answer.

Result

Explain what happened eventually and how it all ended. It is astonishing how many candidates end their answer on a cliff-hanger. There should be a natural resolution to the answer, which ideally results in closure for the patient and the clinical team, with a positive outcome thanks to involvement from yourself as a key player. The answer can then be concluded with a reflection on the scenario and an explanation of the significance of the story to your role as a dentist:

Sample ending

"By recognising the discrepancy, I was able to avoid a potentially serious incident. In addition, this highlighted to me the importance of team working and interfacing effectively with referring clinicians. Finally, the issue of ensuring appropriately informed consent in complex treatment plans is paramount, and I was able to explain things comprehensively to the patient. Having said that, I would have had no hesitation in recommending that we cancel this elective procedure if the patient had not gained a sufficient understanding of the procedure. I highlighted this to the senior clinical staff on duty that day."

One can also summarise skills and learning points demonstrated during the scenario and, in particular, both personal and institutional learning outcomes. The latter consideration commends trainees as likely to make a difference to any unit lucky enough to have them!

Sample ending

"Identifying the shortcomings in this situation made me mindful of the importance of informed consent in modern practice. I take a lot of time to explain treatment plans to patients and, following this, we moved to securing written consent at the initial consultation as a department, as opposed to on the day of surgery, in line with emerging Department of Health guidelines at the time. I also recognised the importance of communicating effectively with referring clinicians and audited our referrals, leading to a standardised orthodontic treatment plan proforma being introduced, which is countersigned by the patient at the initial oral surgery consultation. This has led to a reduction in on-the-day cancellations due to discrepancies in treatment plans and been rated favourably in departmental patient feedback."

5.3 The SPIES structure (for questions on difficult colleagues)

SPIES = Seek information, Patient safety, Initiative, Escalate, Support

Questions asking how you would deal with a difficult colleague come in different shapes and forms. The levels of difficulty vary, from simple lateness to training-related underperformance and attitude problems, to sheer criminal acts. In these questions, the level of seniority of the colleague in question also varies, from a junior clinician to someone more senior, such as a consultant, for example.

This may have implications on how you answer the question, particularly in terms of how able you are going to be to approach the individual concerned directly, what kind of rapport you may have with the person and what kind of formal structures you are going to call on to assist you in raising a concern. This may be partly shaped by the size and nature of departments you have worked in to date; for instance, you may have worked in a maxillofacial department in a district general hospital (DGH) where you knew the two consultants quite well, but this is quite a different beast from a large teaching hospital with 14 consultants, one of whom is the President of the British Association of Oral and Maxillofacial Surgeons (BAOMS)!

Examples of questions frequently asked include:

- "One of your junior colleagues keeps turning up late for clinic and you frequently have to see his/her first patient. What do you do?"
- "What would you do if your consultant came into clinic drunk one morning?"
- "Your consultant is asking you to do something that you feel is wrong, e.g. modifying notes to cover up a mistake. What do you do?"
- "Your registrar constantly fails to answer his/her bleep, leaving you several times in precarious situations. What do you do?"
- "You inadvertently see a sachet of what appears to be cocaine in your registrar's handbag, which is lying open in the staff coffee room. What do you do?"
- "You walk into your consultant's office and see him/her watching images of child pornography on the hospital computer. What do you do?"

The scenarios are daunting and these questions often strike fear into the heart of candidates – most of us imagine the worst case and the thought, for example, of having to remove our drunken boss from the ward. Psychologically, part of the difficulty is to overcome the fear of "what would happen to me if I blew the whistle".

Your interviewers will demand that you understand the broad implications of the scenario, not only for patients, but also for the team and for your colleague. They will be testing your ability to address all the relevant issues appropriately. Having the SPIES structure as a basis for your answer allows you to deal with any of the above questions by applying the same principles.

At the interview, you will be expected to demonstrate that you can handle the situation in a responsible and mature manner, ensuring patient safety at all times, whilst also resolving the matter sensitively.

To ensure that you cover all angles, you will need to consider the following:

Seek information

Before doing anything, you need to ascertain the nature of the issue at hand. The source of the information may be third party (e.g. dental nurses have confided an issue to you concerning your registrar) and there may be hidden agendas and a need for verification. This may involve approaching the individual concerned or another colleague where appropriate, depending upon the gap in seniority between you and the individual concerned, and the rapport you have between you and within the team.

Patient safety

The key issue in all these scenarios will be identifying and addressing patient safety concerns early in the answer. Some patient-safety issues may not be obvious (e.g. coming in late for handover by 20 minutes), but on reflection, you can easily find the issues (e.g. people staying over to cover and being "unsafe", key patient information being missed due to haphazard handover). If the person is an immediate threat (e.g. drunk), you need to remove them from the clinical area. Remember that patient safety may mean retrospectively reviewing and vetting patient encounters (by more senior staff) and ensuring that trust in the team and profession is maintained.

Initiative

Think about whether there is anything you can do to fix things. Only minor issues are likely to be comprehensively addressed by you in isolation, but teams and organisations will always look favourably upon prospective members who demonstrate initiative and, as far as possible, try to resolve things at a local level, provided it is safe to do so.

Escalate

You must involve colleagues at appropriate levels of seniority when required, i.e. when local measures have been unsuccessful or are inappropriate due to the seriousness of the situation/accusation. On the clinical side, this goes up the hierarchy of registrar, consultant, clinical lead, divisional director, etc, etc. From the training point of view, this may be educational supervisor, training programme director, postgraduate dental dean, etc. You should demonstrate an understanding of the hierarchy but at the same time be realistic. If there is a potential criminal issue, involvement of the GDC and authorities may be required.

Support

Remember there are reasons for people acting out, and both the individual and the team/organisation may require support.

This approach is supported by the General Dental Council (GDC) document *Standards for the Dental Team.*

"Standard 8.1
You must always put patients' safety first

8.1.1 You must raise any concern that patients might be at risk due to:

- *the health, behaviour or professional performance of a colleague;*
- *any aspect of the environment where treatment is provided; or*
- *someone asking you to do something that you think conflicts with your duties to put patients interests first and act to protect them*

You must raise a concern even if you are not in a position to control or influence your working environment.

Your duty to raise concerns overrides any personal and professional loyalties or concerns you might have (for example, seeming disloyal or being treated differently by your colleagues or managers)."

"Standard 8.2
You must act promptly if patients or colleagues are at risk and take measures to project them

8.2.1 You must act on concerns promptly. Acting quickly may mean that poor practice is identified and tackled without there being a serious risk to patient safety. If you are not sure whether the issue that worries you amounts to a concern that you should raise, think about what might happen in the short or longer term if you did not mention the issue. If in doubt, you must raise your concern."

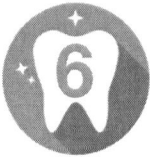

Portfolio station

DCT and ST interviews invariably contain a separate portfolio station, where the interviewers will go through the various sections of the candidate's portfolio and ask relevant questions. In some cases, portfolio stations are merely a formality but, in many others, they are actually a formal station with a formal marking schedule. Either way, the importance of this station should not be underestimated.

Even an informal set-up will involve careful checks of your CV, including any publications or achievements you have listed. As well as any documents you are told to bring, take along evidence of your achievements, including copies of papers or posters (A4 versions are fine). If you are writing or have written a thesis, bring along what you have done – if it is complete, that looks fantastic; if you have written chunks of it, that shows a mark of intent.

Historically, there have been examples of candidates exaggerating their achievements – part of this station's role is to pick that up. It is not unheard of for panels to perform a literature search on candidates – if you are honest, you have nothing to fear, but a lie will fail you that interview and may land you in front of the GDC.

The scoring system varies from specialty to specialty, as well as between deaneries. However, it is commonly as follows:

Oral presentation and communication skills (5 marks)

The candidate will be asked to talk about specific aspects of their experience such as a specific job or rotation. Questions may also be broader; in many portfolio questions, candidates are asked to take the interviewers through their CV or to talk about themselves in no more than two, three or five minutes, depending on the circumstances (see 7.1 and 7.2 for details on how to answer these). Candidates are assessed on their fluency and verbal communication. A lack of structure and coherence, as well as poor eye contact, will usually ensure the lowest mark.

Interaction with the panel (5 marks)

As the panel questions each candidate about their experience, they will be assessing the candidate's ability to consider the questions asked, and the relevance of the answers provided. An ability to think quickly, provide relevant answers and communicate effectively would lead to a high mark, whilst a lack of coherence and relevance would ensure a low mark.

Quality of competence evidence (5 marks)

The panel will be assessing the evidence presented by the candidate to vouch for his/her competence (logbook, DOPs, mini-CEX, etc) and will be judging the organisation, layout, presentation, legibility and completeness of the information. A low score would be given for poor evidence or unclear layout.

Quality of CV (5 marks)

As well as the evidence, the panel will be assessing the quality and layout of the candidate's CV. A comprehensive and well-presented CV with fully relevant information will score highly, whilst a disorganised CV with poor evidence will score low.

The most important bit!

Make sure you lay out your portfolio **exactly** as specified. First, this is an indication of your ability to follow instructions. More importantly, the interviewers will have a limited time with your portfolio to find the items they are scoring. If they cannot find a specific piece of evidence because you have chosen to follow your own layout rather than the one requested, they are well within their rights to withhold marks from you.

There is only one thing more embarrassing than the interviewers not being able to find a piece of evidence in your portfolio, and that is you being unable to locate it! Make sure you know your own portfolio back to front and inside out!

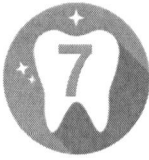

(7) Background & motivation questions

7.1   Take me through your CV

Take me through your CV / Tell me about yourself

This is commonly an opening question in the portfolio station. Whilst in some specialties the portfolio station may be more structured (e.g. in ST1 interviews for oral surgery, candidates were required to focus on two areas of either teaching activity, quality improvement or publication/presentation), in others it is more free (e.g. ST1 orthodontics specifies a "discussion" with the candidate following a review of the candidate's portfolio against a wide range of domains).

Do not literally take them through your CV

This shouldn't be exhaustive and should really be the "highlights". Regard it as a "taster menu" rather than a full meal. Interviewers can pick and choose the areas they want to focus on, and indeed, in many of the dental specialties these will be pre-determined.

Do not worry about overlapping with future questions

Many candidates worry about sounding like a broken record. The advice here would be to treat the question like a table of contents. Also, remember that if there are areas of your experience that you are especially proud of, there is nothing wrong in reinforcing these. You do not know what you might be asked later on in the interview and so you shouldn't be depriving your panel of vital information about you. With separate stations in structured interviews, this is less of an issue, as you may find yourself using the same example to cover multiple dimensions of your professional development, e.g. the international presentation you gave on a quality improvement project might answer a question about clinical governance **and** feature prominently in your response to a generic "Tell me about yourself" question.

Avoid the chronological approach

This can often seem overly lengthy and detailed. As you progress in seniority, things in the distant past seem progressively less relevant. Just as no one is interested in your GCSE results at DFT interviews, the special study module in your BDS degree begins to pale into insignificance at your orthodontics FTTA interview. First, talk about where you are now, working backwards with a broad overview rather than an overly detailed chronology. Remember as well not to dwell on minimum bar points. The panel knows that you have met DCT competencies at an ST1 interview, otherwise you wouldn't be sitting in front of them. They want to know what makes you stand out above your peers.

Apply the CAMP structure

If your CV is well designed, it will likely already be following the CAMP structure. (see 5.1). The same can be said for your portfolio, although it must be stressed that you should follow specialty-specific instructions regarding the layout of your portfolio to the letter. Here is an example of how you could give a general overview of yourself thus far:

Clinical
- Brief chronology of your training (15–20 seconds)
- Description of skills and experience (2–4 points)
- How this motivated you for this specialty

Academic
- Papers you have written
- Relevant postgraduate qualification (or intercalated degrees)
- Postgraduate courses
- Teaching and/or educational qualifications/courses
- Grants you may have won

Management
- Audit experience
- Rota management
- Service development, e.g. implementing changes
- Guidelines/protocols you may have developed
- Committee membership, e.g. DFT/DCT representative
- Event organisation, e.g. BDA study day

Personal
- Personal strengths/skills
- Social life, e.g. achievements, stress release, conducive to region

Sample answer

"My name is John. I am currently a DCT3 in maxillofacial surgery at Worcestershire Royal Hospital. In my current role, I have become proficient at the perioperative care of patients, building upon my prior clinical experience in this specialty at the Queen Elizabeth Hospital in Birmingham. Prior to this, I had DCT placements in paediatric dentistry and orthodontics at the Birmingham Dental Hospital.

"The breadth of experience I have had has given me insights into the challenges faced by the multidisciplinary team charged with the care of orthognathic patients, and I have made a decision to pursue a career in orthodontics. I really enjoy the satisfaction of creating a beautiful smile for patients, working in conjunction with surgical colleagues, and developing a rapport with younger patients and their families.

"I have clinical experience at bond-ups, debonds, treatment planning and removable appliances, including Invisalign, and regularly attend planning clinics for orthognathic patients. My time in paediatric dentistry in particular has made me more aware of the communication challenges with younger patients and their parents, particularly where staged, lengthy treatment plans are required that hinge on good patient cooperation. I have received good feedback from trainers on the clarity of my communication with patients and their relatives, and on my ability to work with a multidisciplinary team in planning treatment commensurate with my current level of training.

"I have developed my teaching skills as well as my clinical skills and have completed a PGCert in dental education. I have arranged a formal teaching programme for medical students at Worcestershire Royal Hospital in oral medicine and early oral cancer diagnosis, which has been well received, and I have received good feedback from students and peer review.

"More recently, I have also developed a new patient information leaflet for skin cancer patients attending the department, as I recognise the importance of written information, to supplement the verbal advice we give to what is often an elderly population. My recent audit in this area highlighted improved patient satisfaction scores and information retention following the introduction of the PIL. My commitment to ensuring that patients are well informed and involved in their care is, in my view, a transferable skill that I can take with me to a career in orthodontics.

"From a more personal perspective, my colleagues see me as someone who is reliable and very supportive. Outside of work, I enjoy team sports such as football and cricket, which give me an outlet to destress. I also enjoy reading and spending time out with friends."

This answer takes approximately two minutes to deliver, at an enthusiastic and engaged pace.

Why this answer works

- It is well structured. You will have recognised that it follows the CAMP structure. The short introduction, where the DCT gives his/her name and his/her current post, is very effective. Obviously, they should already know your name, but the purpose of this sentence is not to provide information. It is designed to build rapport. They won't know you at all, so it is nice to introduce yourself.

- The candidate does not just list information or make bold statements about having experience. It is easy to make statements such as "I have gained a lot of audit and teaching experience", hoping that interviewers might understand what is meant by it. Instead, the candidate provides concrete examples of achievements.

- The candidate recognises that there is no such thing as "bad experience" and uses transferable skills, gained from complementary specialties, in laying the groundwork for being the best "raw material" for higher training in his/her chosen field.

- The candidate ends his/her answer with a more personal slant. Note the use of feedback: "my colleagues see me as someone who is reliable and very supportive." With such a sentence, there is an immediate picture of someone who works well in a team, even though they have never actually said "I am a good team player".

- The information has opened up several avenues of interest that the interviewers can then follow with questions. The information is accurate and punchy – just enough of an appetiser for the panel to gain a feeling of confidence about the candidate.

Ending the answer

Remember to adjust tone of voice to signify a natural end to the answer. Finishing with a personal perspective is good, but a summary of things also works well, e.g.:

> "I feel I am well placed to pursue a career in orthodontics because of my clinical experience, which has laid solid foundations for my career progression, as well as the complementary skills I have developed in clinical governance and research, seeing through lasting changes in any department I work in and providing the best possible care for the patients I treat."

7.2 Tell me about yourself

This question puzzles many candidates, whose first reaction is to ask back, "What do you want me to talk about? Do you want to know about my training, my research, my hobbies?"

If you ask the interviewers to narrow the scope of the question, you will lose a valuable opportunity to demonstrate your full potential. You may also give the impression that you are unable to determine what is important and what is less important to the interviewers, which may then raise questions about your ability to prioritise information.

The purpose of the interview is to determine whether you are the right candidate for the post. Focusing an answer on your hobbies or your personality will not enable you to sell yourself fully. You should aim to tick as many boxes as you can and use the vagueness of the question to your advantage, by presenting your strengths, skills and achievements.

The good news is that, if you have already prepared "Take me through your CV", there is little further preparation to do. Indeed, these two questions are essentially the same, and you can deliver the same answer in exactly the same way.

7.3 Why do you want to train in this specialty?

What the interviewers are looking for

This question is testing your motivation for the post, and the interviewers will be looking for a range of reasons. Marking schedules may take into account some/all of the reasons listed, but commitment to specialty as a whole is often listed in the specialty-specific criteria for selection in many of the dental specialties. If asked the question about commitment to specialty, you should focus on three to four points, ensuring that your reasons are sufficiently different from each other so that you do not sound repetitive and the answer has enough variety to keep the interviewers interested throughout.

Strong explanations with a personal slant are preferred. Make sure your answer is natural, fresh and stands out from the crowd.

Thinking that a specialty suits you is not enough. You should demonstrate that you have tried and tested the role, with either a prior DCT placement or attendance at clinics / treatment sessions, as your schedule permitted. For example, if you were doing a maxillofacial DCT job but are interested in a career in orthodontics, attendance at joint clinics, audits involving orthognathic outcomes and shadowing orthodontic treatment sessions could all be feasible ways of demonstrating interest and commitment.

Remember that these posts are opportunities, and the panel will want to know that you are going to make the most of them. Proving that you have maximised opportunities to date will seal the deal here.

Your choice of specialty needs to come across as something that has been planned. Even if you haven't worked in the field, experience in allied specialties can be seen to equip you with transferable skills and may have been tailored towards your intended career, e.g. having experience in restorative dentistry, oral surgery, orthodontics, public/salaried dental services and/or academic training is a desirable criterion for entry into paediatric dentistry training.

This is not a competition about who will have the best and/or most reasons for entering a given specialty. It is about recruiting those who believe in their future in the specialty. This can only be achieved by talking, in some detail, about what you enjoy. Some of the enthusiasm will be conveyed through your description of your experience to date, but most of it will come from your tone of voice and the enthusiastic manner in which you deliver your answer.

Remember as well that this is about form as well as aspiration. It is about saying as much about why you are suited to a role as it is about why you want to do it. Telling someone you want to be a Formula 1 driver is fine, but you will only be credible if you are able to drive, and have completed two years in junior, single-seater racing events, accumulating race points and mileage requirements in a Formula 1 vehicle!

Defining your reasons for training in the specialty

Avoid statements such as "I find this specialty fascinating" without subsequently defining what you find fascinating about the specialty. Your answers in this regard can be structured around three or four clear reasons, and the CAMP structure (see 5.1) is a useful tool to ensure you cover all the angles. For example:

Clinical reasons
- The technological aspect, e.g. dental radiology
- Interfacing with multiple specialties, e.g. orthodontics
- The "hands-on" aspect, e.g. oral surgery
- The diagnostic dilemmas, e.g. oral medicine
- The fact that it involves prevention as well as treatment, e.g. paediatric dentistry
- Opportunity to work in different settings, e.g. special care dentistry
- Getting immediate results from your work, e.g. oral surgery
- A holistic psychosocial approach, e.g. oral medicine
- Sustained contact with patients over long treatment plans, e.g. orthodontics

Academic reasons
- Fast-advancing specialty with rapidly emerging changes
- Good opportunities for research, e.g. dental public health, periodontology
- Good opportunities for teaching, e.g. oral medicine
- Opportunity to develop a special interest, e.g. dental radiology

Management reasons
- Strong multidisciplinary focus
- Emerging networks requiring strong management responsibility, e.g. MCNs in oral surgery
- Opportunities to develop services and make a real difference to service provision, e.g. Tier 2 contracts in oral surgery
- Preference to work in smaller teams holding greater responsibilities
- Possible scope for regional/national positions as a result of very small specialties, e.g. oral pathology

Personal reasons
- Communication challenges, e.g. special care dentistry
- Dealing with patients in sensitive situations

- Strong influence on patient satisfaction
- Buzz of working under pressure
- Working in an environment where attention to detail matters
- Preference working in larger teams, to learn from a greater variety of people and develop a more sociable environment

The CAMP structure is useful to help you think about a wide range of reasons and gives you a natural structure. You can use it as you see fit in relation to your own situation.

You do not have to find one reason in each category; for example, it would be perfectly fine to have two clinical reasons and one management reason; or one clinical reason, one management reason and one personal reason. What matters is that you can present suitable variety in a structured manner.

It is crucial that you remain true to yourself if you want to appear enthusiastic. Not everyone wants to join a specific specialty for academic reasons, so don't force yourself to talk about academic reasons if they do not represent your true motivations. You will only invite further questions, which will make you regret having mentioned it in the first place.

Ineffective answer

"I have acquired all the fundamental skills to do well in restorative dentistry. I feel I have a lot to offer the specialty. I think the specialty is interesting and rewarding. I like restorative dentistry very much and feel that rehabilitating someone's dentition and occlusion is a truly worthwhile endeavour."

The answer is ineffective because:

- It is principally a list of reasons, with no attempt at substantiation. None of the reasons are explored in any depth, rather the undefined use of words such as "interesting" and "rewarding" makes the answer particularly vacuous. It is unclear what the candidate actually enjoys and why the specialty represents "a worthwhile endeavour".

- The candidate does not attempt to link the points raised to any personal experience or story. The answer, even if developed further, would sound bland and uninteresting, and certainly would not distinguish the candidate from anyone else with the minimum bar qualifications.

- Skills are not a sign of motivation – having the skills to do a job does not necessarily imply the desire to do the work. Dentists generally have restorative skills of varying levels of competence and proficiency, but there is something unique about a career in restorative dentistry *per se* that would tap into the enthusiasm to go above and beyond and develop these further.

The candidate does, however, demonstrate some attempt at the CAMP structure, with an example of a technical reason (e.g. occlusal rehabilitation), a patient-based reason (e.g. the idea of occlusal/restorative rehabilitation being worthwhile) and personal satisfaction.

Effective answer

"Orthodontics is a specialty that I have been passionate about since my undergraduate training, and I sought to explore this passion further and develop a solid foundation to build upon in my dental core training years.

"One aspect I have particularly enjoyed is the multidisciplinary nature of the work. You often interface with other specialties such as maxillofacial surgery, paediatric dentistry and restorative dentistry, in complex treatment plans for patients with hypodontia, for example. I have made efforts to attend and participate in orthognathic planning clinics during my DCT years and saw first-hand how putting many heads together can provide complementary perspectives, to achieve the best outcomes for patients.

"I also love the fact that you can develop a sustained relationship with patients over a lengthy course of treatment. During my DCT placement in the specialty, I got to provide some treatment sessions to the same patients and really enjoyed building a rapport with them and their parents. I enjoyed this, the intellectual challenge of treatment planning and the technical aspects of bond-ups.

"I have enjoyed the fact that the specialty makes a difference to patients' confidence levels, and I helped gather data for a national audit into PROMs for orthognathic surgery. There is an advancing research side to the specialty as well, and I was also fortunate enough to be involved with a project looking at the role of simulation software in predicting outcomes in orthognathic surgery.

"From a personal perspective, orthodontics involves manual dexterity and mental agility in equal measure. I feel I have the fundamentals in terms of clinical, academic and management experience to date, to grab the opportunities offered in higher training."

The answer demonstrates personal enthusiasm, form as well as aspiration, and awareness of multiple facets to the role and due respect for higher training as an opportunity to be maximised.

Beware of criticising other specialties

Many of the dental specialties state categorically that experience in other specialties is a desirable quality in a candidate. Be very careful about criticising other specialties. For instance, oral surgery candidates might perceive orthodontics as having lengthy treatment plans, which are slow to achieve results and therefore "boring" or very "monotonous", whilst oral surgery yields immediate outcomes. Conversely, orthodontists may regard oral surgeons as having no patience or willingness to develop a rapport with patients over a long time period.

You can see how inflammatory such answers can be. Ultimately, interviewers will be looking to see that you can identify the learning points in any job you do and the transferable skills you bring with you. Skills in managing challenging aspects of patient compliance or cooperation, in community dental jobs or paediatric dentistry DCT time, will serve you well in just about any other clinical role. There will be high and low points to any specialty training programme, and aspects of the training that will test your resolve and commitment due to wavering interest. Not being able to recognise the value in a breadth of dental foundation and core training placements will call into question your ability to see through a varied higher-training programme.

Above and beyond the inability to identify transferable skills, criticism of other specialties generally paints you in a negative light, and the comment "I wonder what he/she will say about us to the next group of people" may well be asked after you leave the interview room!

If you have made a leap from one specialty to another and changed career path (e.g. leaving a specialty training job), then this is the only exception to the rule. In this instance, it would be acceptable to explain your interest in your new specialty of choice with reference to your previous specialty, comparing the two. If you do this, you still need to make sure that you set out the positive points of your previous specialty. When mentioning the negative aspects, present them as something that you did not enjoy, rather than generalising with sentences like "Specialty <xxx> is not very interesting because ...".

The best format to explain a switch of specialty would be to explain:
- What you enjoyed about your previous specialty
- Why you felt limited within it
- Why this new specialty is the answer to your problems

Selling your enthusiasm for a dental core training (DCT) post

Those who are applying to named specialties (e.g. restorative dentistry, oral surgery, paediatric dentistry) may find it easier to explain their career choices than those applying to generic DCT posts. This particularly applies for those applying to oral and maxillofacial surgery DCT posts, as in all honesty, these are often pursued secondary to perceived "more desirable" but less available DCT posts in dental hospitals, by candidates looking to pursue higher training in dental specialties rather than a career in oral and maxillofacial surgery *per se*.

There are, however, properties common to all dental specialties and maxillofacial surgery, and it is worth thinking about transferable skills between specialties:

Good interpersonal skills
Challenging situations may be encountered in patients with learning difficulties in community / special care dentistry, younger patients in paediatric dentistry, and drunk/aggressive patients in maxillofacial surgery. The transferable skills are similar in modifying interaction to achieve the best possible care.

Time management
You can be working under pressure in a busy maxillofacial on call, but equally, keeping to time in practice requires meticulous planning!

Prioritisation
You might prioritise unwell patients in your maxillofacial job but also when facing a paediatric dentistry emergency / dental trauma clinic.

Teamwork
Inter-specialty and multidisciplinary working can be seen in every job. Think about the teams making up cleft patient care, facial deformity clinics, hypodontia clinics. You may be on any of these teams but still see the full remit of what each has to offer and how they work together. An essential transferable skill.

Technical skills
Manual dexterity is required in many dental specialties. Placing a disto-occlusal amalgam in an upper second molar may equip you with excellent skills for taking out a wisdom tooth!

Others may include evidence-based practice, dealing with the unexpected, the breadth and variety of work encountered, and we are sure you can think of more! By following a similar pattern to the answer given earlier and, more importantly, by using your own experience, you will be able to create a strong answer.

If you already have an idea of the specialty you wish to do once you have completed your DCT training, then we would suggest that you use it in your answer too. However, be careful to only bring it up at the end of the answer. If you go on about one single specialty throughout the whole answer, you will cause three problems:

- The consultants interviewing you may be from a different specialty and will be looking for some balance (you wouldn't want to bruise their egos too much!)
- You will give the feeling that you may be bored during the DCT rotation whenever you are not working in your chosen specialty. This could be problematic if you are given a DCT rotation outside of your chosen specialty.
- You could potentially be setting yourself up for questions about what you will do if you don't secure your chosen specialty at the end of DCT rotations.

In addition, dentistry is a small world. You may find yourself working for the person who interviewed you, and there would inevitably be some preconceptions if you had expressed no interest in specialty X.

By spending time talking about dentistry in general and the generic competencies and skills you hope to acquire from dental core training, whilst focusing on your chosen specialty in the final paragraph, you will establish a sensible balance in your answer. This will show that you are motivated for the whole programme but that you also have a clear focus.

Better still, you could identify two specialties of a similar nature. For example, paediatric dentistry and special care dentistry both have challenges in terms of communication with patients and tailoring explanations to different audiences, as well as dealing with third parties (e.g. parents, carers). By mentioning the two specialties rather than one, you also present yourself as someone who is open minded.

So, your final paragraph could run:

"Finally, the two specialties that I have particularly enjoyed have been paediatric dentistry and special care dentistry. They present challenges in terms of seeing through treatment plans and involving parents and/or carers in gaining patients' trust and compliance, as well as demanding optimal communication with patients and their families. I enjoy the challenge of this and the sense of satisfaction in achieving the best possible care for these patient groups, under what can at times be challenging conditions. I would like to get more experience of both specialties in my DCT years, so that I can make the right choice for my higher training."

7.4 What is your biggest achievement?

This is a question that gives you the opportunity to impress. The question says "biggest", so stick to one achievement. Mentioning more than one achievement would only dilute the strength of your answer, because you would talk superficially about several rather than in-depth about one. You would also be wasting time, because the marking scheme will only allow you to score points for one achievement.

This question is not very specific as to what type of achievement the interviewers are looking for. You have a choice between achievements within dentistry or outside dentistry, academic achievements or non-academic achievements, etc. If you have one particular achievement that you are keen on highlighting, mention that one. If you have several and are unsure as to which they would prefer, then you can ask them what type of achievement they are looking for.

Deriving content for your answer

Use the **CAMP** structure (see 5.1) to help you derive possible achievements:

Clinical
- Breadth of experience gained
- Progression in training over expectations
- Initiative taken to gain experience in your specialty of choice well beyond basic training requirements
- Prizes or awards at dental school or during your postgraduate training

Academic
- Substantial involvement in a research project
- Substantial involvement in teaching
- Involvement in the preparation and delivery of an important presentation
- Publication of paper, audit, poster or case report, preferably as first author
- Prize for presentation or poster
- Teaching achievements or recognition, e.g. developing in-house teaching in a practice such as BLS, IRMER or sedation training

Management
- Substantial involvement in audit, or taking charge of an audit that led to important changes in clinical practice
- Successful management of a rota for a complex team or set-up
- Writing a guideline or protocol

Personal

- Voluntary work or out-of-programme experience (OOPE)
- Position of responsibility outside of dentistry
- Implementing educational website or other key resource
- Having successfully juggled training with difficult personal circumstances
- High achievement in sports, music, arts, etc

Marking scheme

Marking schemes may vary, but they will always centre around the strength of the achievement and the explanation of its significance to you. A typical marking scheme would be as follows:

0	No real achievement
1	Moderate achievement with reasonable explanation of significance
2	High achievement with reasonable explanation of significance, or Moderate achievement with clear, detailed explanation of significance
3	Exceptional achievement with reasonable explanation of significance, or High achievement with clear, detailed explanation of significance
4	Exceptional achievement with clear, detailed explanation of significance

Nature and strength of the achievement

To produce an effective answer, you must explain clearly not only what the achievement is, but also why it is an achievement. This will help the interviewers to mark it as moderate, high or exceptional. The following table is often used by interviewers to determine the level of the achievement:

Exceptional	Less than 10% of your peers would be expected to achieve the same thing, or there was a high level of competition.
High	Less than 25% of your peers would be expected to achieve the same thing, or there was a reasonable level of competition.
Moderate	Less than 50% of your peers would be expected to achieve the same thing, or there was some competition.

You will greatly help the interviewers to mark you well by ensuring that you define how hard you needed to work in order to achieve your goal and/or the level of competition that you faced.

Explanation of the achievement's significance to you

This is an important part of the answer, which is often neglected by candidates. The interviewers will not only want to know that you can achieve; they will also want you to demonstrate that you understand the significance of your achievement and what it says about you. In your answer, you should therefore highlight why you are particularly proud of your achievement and what can be derived from it. You will also need to make the link back to the post or specialty that you are applying for.

Example 1: **Dental school prize**

Saying "I received a prize at dental school in the human disease module" does not reflect accurately the level of the achievement. The interviewer will not know how hard you needed to work to obtain it or how much competition you faced. Instead, you will need to say something along the following lines:

Achievement: "My biggest achievement is a prize that I obtained at dental school in the human disease module. I was competing against 72 other students. I secured the highest marks in the written component of the examination. I was then invited to a prize viva, where I was quizzed by a panel of examiners on the clinical applications of the knowledge we had acquired in the module, working through some challenging simulated cases. It involved a lot of preparation, which I had essentially done throughout the year in reading around the topics we covered and going deeper in my understanding. In addition, I paid close attention to clinical encounters on my placement in a district general hospital, to see how the lectures were clinically relevant.

Significance: "I am particularly proud of the prize because I worked hard to ensure that I was well prepared for the assessment, and the reward reflects the interest that I paid to the module. It validated my ability to apply knowledge and to understand a breadth of knowledge outside of practical dentistry, which I hope will prepare me well for a career in maxillofacial surgery, as well as in caring for patients holistically, a consideration ever more important in the face of an aging population with increasingly complex comorbidities."

This answer is effective because both the level of the achievement and effort required are clearly set out by the candidate. The explanation of the significance is also well developed. The candidate demonstrates why they were proud of the achievement and what it meant to them.

Example 2: **Poster presentation**

If you consider the answer "During one of my attachments, we had a poster accepted at a regional conference, for which we nearly got a prize", you will see that the impact is minimal. The achievement itself seems exceptional for someone at DFT level; however, the lack of explanation, coupled with the fact that the candidate talks about "we", i.e. the team rather than him-/herself, makes it difficult to mark. A better answer would be as follows:

Achievement: "During my DCT1 year in paediatric dentistry, I conducted an audit on pain relief in alveolar bone grafting in cleft palate patients. The audit highlighted some severe issues, which I summarised in a presentation to my department, following which I was encouraged to write up the audit results as a poster presentation for the BAOMS conference. Not only was my poster accepted for exhibition, it was also selected for an oral presentation, which I gave, and for which I received a BAOMS members prize.

Significance: "I am very proud of this achievement for several reasons. First, I played a leading role in the audit and was able to point out some severe failures of the system, which ultimately led to a change in practice and improved patient care. Secondly, being selected for a poster presentation was my first major academic achievement, but being asked to do the presentation really gave me pride in my work. Finally, I was able to put together a good presentation with very little notice, and, although I did not get the first prize, I came close, and it really motivated me to get further involved in audits and studies so that I can do even better next time."

This answer works well because we can easily identify the level of involvement and effort made by the candidate. There is sufficient detail, without it being boring to listen to (for example, the actual results of the audit were missed out deliberately because, by themselves, they do not form part of the achievement – if the interviewers were interested in the results, they could always ask further questions). The significance of the achievement is also very well laid out, with a good explanation of the motivation gained by the candidate as a result of it.

7.5 What do you like most about this specialty?

The answer to this question can be taken directly from question 7.3 – "Why do you want to train in this specialty?" – as they are effectively the same question. It may be, however, that the interviewers ask you to focus on one specific positive point of the specialty. You can simply pick on one of the points, but this may leave you with a feeling that you are not selling yourself fully. There is a good trick that you can adopt if you want to present several attributes in the same answer, without sounding like you are not answering the question properly. Consider this answer:

> "There are plenty of aspects that I like about paediatric dentistry. I enjoy the teamwork element of the specialty, the communication challenge of having to convey similar information at child and adult levels, as well as the fact that you can deal with a lot of specialties within the course of one day.
>
> "However, if I had to isolate one particular aspect of paediatric dentistry, I would say that what I enjoy most is that you can really make a strong difference to someone's life, and there is nothing that gives me more satisfaction than the smile on a mother's face when she sees that we have made a big difference to her child. It can be very emotional but it is also very rewarding at times. For example, <then talk briefly about a recent situation that illustrates your point>."

If you look closely at the answer, you will see that the candidate has mentioned briefly a few positive features of the specialty, before quickly settling on what he/she regards as the most rewarding. In all fairness, the marking scheme is likely to account only for one positive, and therefore, as such, you may not score extra marks for the daring introduction. However, this technique will make your answer much more dynamic. In turn, it will make you sound more enthusiastic, and it may well influence the interviewers subconsciously in providing a slightly higher mark. This could be the difference between getting three marks for a good answer and four marks for an excellent answer.

7.6 What do you like least about this specialty?

The interviewers will be looking for honesty and a realistic insight into the specialty. Here are some examples of points that you can raise:

- Oral medicine: being given inappropriate referrals
- Oral surgery: some aspects of the work may be repetitive
- Paediatric dentistry: it can be emotionally difficult to deal with cases where you know that there is little you can do for a child; dealing with challenging child protection issues
- Oral and maxillofacial surgery: having to put up with angry or drunk patients or the feeling that sometimes you are dealing with things outside of your comfort zone!
- Dental and maxillofacial radiology: a lot of solo work (e.g. reporting); having to fight unreasonable requests from other specialists
- Dental public health: lack of patient contact; distance from clinical environment and "front line"
- Special care dentistry: protection issues; patchy provision of services; patients "falling through the gaps" in the system
- Endodontics: inappropriate referrals; unrealistic expectations of patients; "herodontics"
- Oral and maxillofacial pathology: distance from clinical environment and lack of patient contact; issues with training pathway and overlap with medically qualified pathologists; peer perception
- Oral microbiology: limitations of a small specialty for networking and collaborating
- Periodontology: unrealistic expectations; inappropriate referrals

There are no right or wrong answers. However, in order to optimise the impact of your answer, you will need to consider the following:

- Unless specifically asked, do not mention more than one negative aspect.
- You must justify your answer using your experience.
- If you can, introduce your answer with one or two quick positive aspects, to place the negative into a more neutral context.
- Reassure the interviewers that you can deal/cope with this negative, and explain how/why.

Example of an effective answer

Positive introduction	"I find it difficult to find something that I don't like in special care dentistry because I think that the specialty has a lot to offer, both in terms of variety and the personal satisfaction to be able to deal with people who are particularly vulnerable; however, this is not without its own challenges.
Clear answer	"There is perhaps one aspect of special care dentistry that I have enjoyed less than others, and this is the fact that we sometimes have to deal with patients with comorbidities, who may have been better managed in a hospital setting but, by virtue of an overstretched system, are being cared for in the community. The difficulty in interfacing with the acute hospital trusts can be frustrating.
Illustrative example	"For example, a couple of months ago, during my special care dentistry placement, I dealt with a patient who had a rare immunodeficiency syndrome and had developed a facial swelling. It was presumed to be an odontogenic infection, and the patient had been told to attend by the local maxillofacial department, but it was readily apparent that this was a chronic sinusitis, which had an acute 'flare-up'. I had to contact the patient's GP, who had an overbooked clinic that day; and I then had to interface with the hospital department, who had wrongly attributed the patient's complain to a dental source.
Coping with it	"I am usually very good at dealing with pressure, and I have always been able to handle the more 'hairy' moments appropriately and with good outcomes. One of the reasons I want to do special care dentistry is the ability to make a difference to vulnerable patients, and to help 'plug the gaps' in a system of care that often relies on the informal contribution from general dental practitioners, who may not have the benefits of specialty training or the time to develop a special interest in looking after what can be complex and daunting issues in challenging patients."

7.7 What have you done outside of your regular scheduled daily activities that demonstrates your interest in the specialty?

The question is asking for experience that you organised to gain an insight into the specialty. Note that the question precludes you from discussing any activities that formed part of your normal duties. It has to be above your normal duties, i.e. something that you took the initiative to organise or to get involved in.

Finding content for your answer

The list below contains some of the experiences that you can use to sell your interest and commitment:

- Seeking special attachments or "tasters" in the specialty
- Attending relevant teaching sessions
- Undertaking a project in the specialty (e.g. audits, presentations)
- Discussing a possible career in the specialty with a consultant
- Shadowing an DCT/ST in your spare time
- Voluntarily sitting in on clinics in that specialty
- Reading up on specialty-related issues (journals, internet sites)
- Attending conferences (specialty associations or other)
- Studying for exams or certificates related to the specialty
- Online CPD activities through recognised institutions/websites
- Choosing an elective at dental school that was in that field
- Doing a dissertation for your intercalated BSc, or otherwise on a related topic

Think laterally about experience acquired in related specialties

The experience does not have to be in the specialty itself. For example, let's assume that you wanted to apply to orthodontics. One obvious way to demonstrate your interest in the specialty would be to initiate an audit during an orthodontics attachment. However, you may also have used your initiative to get involved in orthodontics-related projects during DFT in your dental practice, during DCT in maxillofacial surgery or via hypodontia clinics in restorative dentistry.

Similarly, if you are applying for oral surgery, you may have volunteered to attend additional theatre sessions during your maxillofacial surgery placement, carrying out dentoalveolar procedures. You may also have attended specialist clinics in the hypodontia team as part of your paediatric dentistry placement, interfacing with the specialty.

Marking schedule

A typical marking schedule would be as follows:

0	No clear evidence
1	Examples are not related to the specialty, or they are, but the candidate has not demonstrated the relevance
2	Some evidence provided but it is basic, explanations are relatively vague and relevance to the specialty is not explained
3	One good example provided with relevance to the specialty highlighted, clear explanation of how the candidate developed experience, skills or understanding as a result
4	More than one good example provided, showing relevance to the specialty, clearly explaining how the candidate developed their experience, skills or understanding as a result

From this sample marking schedule, you can clearly see that, to maximise your mark, you need to provide several relevant examples with full explanation of relevance and personal reflection. Any vagueness in the answer will make you score at most two marks, even if you have several items to discuss.

Example of an effective answer (dental and maxillofacial radiology)

"In addition to my regular discussions with dental radiologists in the course of all my previous jobs, whether they were in the emergency dental clinics, paediatric dentistry or restorative dentistry, I have also sought many additional opportunities to become involved in dental and maxillofacial radiology audit projects or studies, and completed two projects last year, under the guidance of a consultant radiologist.

"I performed an audit on the quality of radiographs in my DFT practice and did a study that compared sialendoscopy with sialography. Both enabled me to get a good grasp of some of the important issues affecting radiology, particularly on the interventional side.

"I have also made every effort to attend courses that would enhance my knowledge. Over the past two years, I have attended four radiology-related courses, on topics as diverse as IRMER updates and minimally invasive techniques in obstructive salivary gland disease. I am due to attend a further meeting later this year on plain film reporting. Although some of these courses were quite complex, they provided me with a better understanding of some of the issues that I had come across during my previous posts. They have also shown me the diversity that dental and maxillofacial radiology offers.

"Finally, I have taken up membership of the British Society of Dental and Maxillofacial Radiology. This gives me access to a range of websites and publications, which I consult in my spare time. Like the courses that I attend, it gives me further insight into the specialty. Some of the sites also have online CPD exercises, which I have found useful."

Example of an effective answer (oral surgery)

"Oral surgery is the specialty that I have most enjoyed over the past few years and, as a result, I have taken the initiative to get involved in many projects in this field.

"I have recently attended the BAOS annual conference and regularly attend junior trainee meetings, as well as a regional study group. I found these events to be an excellent complement to my daily activities, as they allow me to continue to touch base with the specialty, whilst training in other complementary dental specialties in my DCT years, but also allow me to consolidate what I learn on the shop floor.

"On top of that, I have made a point of attending several oral surgery courses. Over the past three years, I have attended an average of three courses per year, including a modular course on oral implantology at the Eastman. These courses have helped me in my daily work, and proactively getting involved in continuing professional development will put me in good stead to keep my skills up to date throughout my career.

"Finally, I have attended the optional weekly oral surgery journal club within my own institution, and combined oral surgery / restorative dentistry meetings, to discuss complex multidisciplinary cases. These have been particularly useful in helping me understand the interaction between oral surgery and other specialties, and certainly showed me how much more can be achieved through teamwork, even when there are disagreements."

Example of an effective answer (oral microbiology)

"During my DCT placement in oral medicine last year, I arranged to sit in on a number of oral microbiology laboratory sessions with the local consultant oral microbiologist. I watched laboratory technicians at work, reporting sessions, and the consultant interfacing with other specialties, which gave me an excellent insight into the nature of the clinical problems encountered as well as of the intricacies of managing patients with oral microbiology issues. In particular, I gained an appreciation of the interface with other specialties.

"Last year I did an audit of needle stick injuries amongst hospital staff. Through this audit, I learnt much about risk management and the prescription of post-exposure prophylaxis. It also gave me an opportunity to discover how A&E handles occupational injuries. This was complementary to my understanding of the clinical relevance of microbiology in general, and how it impacts on other specialties and institutions as a whole.

"Finally, I have attended two conferences, one on the impact of periodontitis and the oral microbiome on cardiovascular health, and the other on the importance of early recognition of herpes zoster in prevention of post-herpetic neuralgia, which gave me a good introduction to current issues."

All three examples work well because they contain three key points, which are developed in a personal manner. The candidate sticks to the point and avoids waffling. This makes the delivery confident and enables the interviewers to tick the boxes.

7.8   Where do you see yourself in 10 years' time?

This question requires some degree of thought if you don't want to provide an answer of the type "Well, I see myself as a consultant caring for patients", which would be quoting the obvious and would guarantee you a poor mark. Again, you can think along the lines of the CAMP structure (see 5.1), to gather your thoughts and structure your answer:

Clinical
- If you are applying for a dental core training scheme, which specialty would you like to get into? There is no need to focus on one if you can't, but try to narrow your preferences a little to your most likely choices.
- If you are applying for a specific specialty, are there any particular interests that you want to develop? For example, if you are applying for ST1 oral medicine, would you be more interested by facial pain, vesiculobullous disorders, joint work with dermatology – what is your unique selling point (USP)? If you are applying for restorative dentistry, perhaps you are interested in implantology, cleft lip and palate patients, or the role of restorative dentistry in the rehabilitation of oral cancer patients.
- You clearly want to be a specialist, but do you want to be community-based, or do you want to pursue post-specialism training to enable you to take up a consultant role within the specialty?

Academic
- Are you interested in doing research? If so, why? What makes you say that? Do you already have experience of research? What topics interest you?
- Have you already developed research interests that you are keen to pursue?
- Do you have an interest in teaching, which you are keen to develop? What kind of personal development do you envisage undertaking? Do you want to be involved in training the next generation of specialists and/or undergraduate students? Do you want to get involved at royal college level? Are there particular areas that you have enjoyed teaching and would like to become further involved in? Do you intend to gain further teaching qualifications (e.g. medical education degree)?

Management
- Do you want to be involved in service development? Perhaps you have had opportunities to get involved in developing guidelines or improving services, e.g. oral surgery managed clinical networks (MCNs)
- Are you interested in managing and supervising others, for example by becoming an educational supervisor?
- Are you interested in developing training programmes?

- Do you have an interest in some aspects of governance, in which you would like to become involved (e.g. patient information, risk management)?
- In 10 years' time, you won't have had a chance to become clinical director, but you could look slightly further and determine whether you are keen to develop management responsibilities further down the line.

Personal

- Which type of region do you see yourself working in?
- What type of team do you see yourself being part of?
- Responsibilities outside work (e.g. charity, voluntary work)
- Hobbies

Example of an effective answer (for ST1 restorative dentistry)

"10 years is a long way away but, certainly by that time, I will have completed my training and become a consultant. So far, I have particularly enjoyed working in dental hospital settings, because you are often dealing with a lower turnover of more complex patients and with a wide spectrum of problems. This is therefore the setting in which I see myself working in the long term. Clinically, I will have the opportunity, through my specialty training, to determine which subspecialty area of interest I enjoy most; however, so far, I have particularly enjoyed the oral rehabilitation of head and neck cancer patients. There is a satisfaction element relating to the complex treatment planning, working with other specialties and a potential research component that could form part of my future practice.

"Over the past couple of years, I have really enjoyed participating in teaching programmes. I gave lectures to dental students, I ran revision workshops for finals and even mentored juniors and students on the job. This is certainly an avenue that I am keen to develop; and to achieve this, I am keen to attend a number of teaching courses and perhaps also do a medical education degree. I know that these degrees can be quite time-consuming and I therefore think it would be a good idea if I started doing it earlier in my career, rather than when I get too close to my IFSE and CCST dates, to give it the time it deserves. From a more personal perspective, I am involved outside of work in voluntary work, teaching disadvantaged children at a local school and raising funds for a charity, which sends medical equipment to African countries, and I would hope that I get sufficient time to continue my involvement with either these institutions or others of a similar nature."

This answer works well because:

- It goes beyond the obvious and demonstrates that the candidate has put some thought into his/her career and motivation.
- It has three points clearly signposted and expanded upon.
- It covers a range of activities (clinical, teaching, voluntary work).

Note also the nice touch brought into the answer by the recognition that doing a medical education degree is hard work (in fact many people give up before they complete them). It is this type of sentence that clearly demonstrates that the candidate has done his/her homework.

7.9   What skills do you need to improve?

It would be easy to provide an answer such as "I feel that my training has been excellent so far and there is therefore nothing that I need to improve". However, this would score low because, in actual fact, the question aims to determine whether you have any insight into your own skills and attributes, and whether you are proactive in seeking ways to improve. Importantly, the question does not refer to new skills that you want to gain in future, but to existing skills that you need to improve. The distinction is important if you want to avoid going off topic.

Brainstorming for ideas

To think about different topics that you could raise, use the CAMP structure (see 5.1):

Clinical
- Are there procedures that you need to perfect?
- Did you miss out on opportunities to develop exposure to some conditions or procedures, either because you were busy building other parts of your CV or because the departments in which you rotated did not have a sufficient number of patients on whom you could train?
- Are there areas of clinical practice that could be consolidated or improved, by going to formal courses or attending special clinics?

Academic
- Have you been involved in research and struggled with some aspects of it? Perhaps you have not done any research yet, have gained research-related skills on an ad hoc basis, and want to formalise your learning?
- Have you got any teaching experience and want to develop certain aspects of it? Are there aspects of teaching or presentation skills that you need to improve (e.g. speaking to large audiences, or learning to make your teaching sessions more interactive)?

Management
- Did you wish you had done more audits?
- Did you miss out on management opportunities such as organising rotas?
- Have you found it hard sometimes to deal with the complexity of project management?
- Have you found it difficult to negotiate your way out of difficult situations and need to develop more confidence (e.g. interfacing with other specialties with conflicting viewpoints on patient management)?

- Have you found it difficult to find your place in multidisciplinary meetings, and that you need to gain more confidence and assertiveness?

Personal
- Are there interpersonal skills in which you wish you could have had more formal training?

Answering the question

There is no need to be too negative about your training. You must be proud of whatever you have done so far and be honest about your areas of weakness. Overall, you want to convey that everything went well, but that there are some minor areas that you could have handled differently.

The answer could be structured as follows:
- Explain that you really enjoyed your training and why.
- State clearly the area that you feel could have been handled differently.
- Explain how you feel you should have handled it.
- Explain how you plan to correct this in the forthcoming years.

Example of an effective answer

"I feel that my training to date has been extremely good. As well as developing good clinical practice and judgement, I have also built a good portfolio of audits, teaching experience and research exposure, including one publication. The one area that I feel I have not had much opportunity to develop is my management skills. Although I have been involved in a number of projects, such as <x, y and z>, where I was able to demonstrate good leadership, I feel that the lack of formal management training and the fact that we constantly rotate between jobs makes it difficult to consolidate all the skills learnt on the job.

"I have tried to counter this by having discussions and informal training with my educational supervisor, but I would benefit more by being involved in more long-term projects and attending formal training. As soon as I start my ST1 training, I plan to raise the issue with my consultants so that I can plan my career well ahead in that respect. I would hope to improve this by continuing my interest at work and by attending an appropriate management course."

Another example of an effective answer

"During the course of my training so far, I have been heavily developing my audit and teaching portfolio, which has enabled me to learn an awful lot about service improvement, training and communication skills. However, as a result, I have not had much time to undertake research work. I know that, as a trainee, it is important to develop research skills in order to understand the evidence that we base our practice on. As such, I am keen to develop my understanding of research further. I plan to achieve this by attending and organising journal clubs, but also by enrolling myself on courses on topics such as research methodologies. I am also keen to write and publish a paper in my next job."

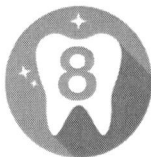

8 Skills-based questions

Skills-based questions form a substantial part of the bank of those asked at interviews. They can take the form of asking about generic personal attributes such as communication, leadership skills and team playing. They often also require you to provide specific examples where you demonstrated these skills.

Most candidates tend to neglect these questions during their preparation for interviews, either because they feel they can "wing it", or because they are unsure as to how the questions should be approached, preferring instead to bury their head in the sand, hoping that some of the awkward questions such as "What is your main weakness?" won't come up. The scores on these questions more commonly reflect this lack of preparation – therefore, this represents a real opportunity for you to gain points that will separate you from the crowd.

In truth, generic questions can be very difficult to handle at an interview if you have not thought your answers through prior to the big day. We would, therefore, encourage you to spend some time organising your thoughts on the matters raised in this chapter.

8.1 How would you describe your communication skills?

What communication skills are they looking for?

The interviewers will be looking for an answer that is mature, relevant to the specialty that you are applying for and backed up with personal examples. To score highly, you must present different facets of your communication skills, demonstrate their relevance to the specialty and provide suitable examples.

Communication is an integral part of your daily working life and is the cement that ensures that you maintain good relationships and that you are effective in your work. In the course of your work, you generally demonstrate the following communication skills:

> **Active listening and empathy**
>
> Active listening and empathy are ways of letting the other person know that you understand their feelings, that you care about what they are saying and that you are non-judgemental.
>
> In your dealings with others, this will translate into the following behaviours:
>
> - Knowing when to keep silent and let the other person speak
> - Not interrupting
> - Being attentive to what the other person is saying and showing it (open posture, appropriate nodding and good eye contact)
> - Probing in a supportive manner and using open questions
> - Showing support, warmth, care and attention
> - Being sensitive to the emotions of others
>
> You can demonstrate such behaviours in the following situations:
>
> - Breaking bad news
> - Talking to an upset patient, relative or colleague
> - Dealing with an angry person (patient or colleague)
> - Handling complaints
> - Dealing with a conflict
> - Discussing problems with colleagues (work-related or personal)

As a result, you will achieve the following:

- Gain cooperation from the other person
- Build trust and develop rapport
- Make people feel more confident
- Encourage discussion and greater openness

You may also reflect on the fact that you learn the generic skill of conveying information in a clear and structured manner to a variety of audiences (patients and peers) as a dentist in postgraduate training.

Conveying information in a clear and structured manner

As a dentist, you need to convey your message in a manner that suits your audience. In practice, this will include the following behaviours:

- Anticipating the needs of your audience
- Using clear and unambiguous language, with appropriate jargon
- Choosing the most appropriate communication method, e.g. written, face to face, telephone, email, models, diagrams, leaflets
- Adapting your communication to the understanding of your audience

You can demonstrate such behaviours in the following situations:

- Explaining procedures or management plans to patients
- Seeking consent
- Writing treatment plans, reports or notes
- Presenting a patient to a senior colleague, with a view to gaining advice
- Teaching colleagues
- Presenting at a meeting
- Educating a patient about a chronic condition
- Constructing patient information leaflets (PILs)
- Giving lifestyle / oral hygiene advice

As a result, you will achieve the following:

- Better cooperation and appropriate response from the other person
- Time efficiency
- Fewer mistakes/errors

Your day-to-day role may also involve some key negotiating skills in interacting with allied health professionals / other dental professionals, and other medical and dental specialties. You may be confronted with difficult situations, disagreements or event conflicts. To resolve these situations, you will need to influence other people (i.e. make sure that they do what you believe to be in the best interests of the patient, without coercing/manipulating others, which could aggravate conflicts and build resentment in a team).

Influencing and negotiating skills

- Understanding the impact of your communication on others and adapting your approach accordingly
- Confidently but non-aggressively setting out and defending your point of view
- Being tactful and diplomatic
- Being encouraging and constructive when talking to others

You can demonstrate such behaviours in the following situations:

- Dealing with a difficult colleague (e.g. one not pulling his/her weight)
- Dealing with difficult patients or complaints
- Conflicts with nurses or allied health professionals / dental professionals
- Conflict within a multidisciplinary environment, due to different personal agendas
- Negotiating the referrals of a patient from a community/dental hospital to an acute hospital
- Designing rotas/timetables
- Negotiating study or annual leave

As a result, you will achieve:

- Outcomes that match your expectations
- Better working relationships with and understanding of your colleagues

---

Answering the question

To produce an effective answer, you need to reflect on your day-to-day experiences and determine in which context you have used the above skills. You only need to discuss a small number of points, but it is important that these points are backed up by your personal experience. The answer must be *your* answer and not some standard explanation of what constitutes communication skills. Blow your own trumpet. At an interview, you must sell yourself positively; it would make no sense to play down your communication skills. Even if you think that you are not that good, you need to find the courage to state that you are; if you don't sell yourself, the interviewers won't be doing it for you! Phrases to avoid:

- "My communication skills are above average" (not very positive)
- "My communication skills are okay" (meaningless and uninspiring)
- "My communication skills could be improved" (are they bad?)
- "I would give myself 8 out of 10 (meaningless – why not 9 or 10?)
- "I think that I have good communication skills", if delivered in a sceptical voice (if delivered confidently, it could be okay)
- "My communication skills are excellent" (don't overdo it!)
- "My English could be improved" (they will be testing your English at the interview – no need to shoot yourself in the foot by reminding them of a potential weakness)
- "I am a good communicator because I can speak five languages" (the fact that you can speak several languages doesn't mean that you can communicate; there are plenty of people who speak English perfectly and are not good communicators. Of greater relevance would be your ability to relate to people at different levels, including those from other cultures or ethnic backgrounds. Languages are only tools that help you achieve this).

Good phrases to use:

- "I have good communication skills"
- "My communication skills are very good"
- "I have developed good communication skills" (this recognises that communication is an evolving skill)
- "I have effective communication skills" (meaning that they are achieving results – it saves you having to say that you are good)
- "I have received very positive feedback on my communication skills, not only from nurses and other colleagues, but also from patients" (Remember: feedback is a good way to introduce objectivity in your answers)

Many candidates feel uneasy saying that they are good. This unease comes from the tendency to limit their answer to a single statement of the type "I feel that I have good communication skills" which, if not backed up by concrete examples, will sound very boastful and arrogant. Your answers can sound genuine only if you mention practical examples; by being down to earth and practical, you will reach your comfort zone, which in turn will make you feel more confident in your delivery. Mentioning feedback received will also help make your answers more realistic and will make you sound and feel more confident.

> **Example of an ineffective answer**
>
> "I think that my communication skills are okay but obviously can be improved. Communication is particularly important in my specialty because we have to discuss complex treatment plans with patients and be able to talk to them in a way they understand. We also have to deal with difficult or uncooperative patients and work with other specialties. I can speak several languages, including English, Polish and Italian, which can be extremely useful in the region where I work. I have also done quite a bit of teaching, which is important in my specialty."

Whilst there is an attempt to discuss a variety of communication issues, the answer comes up short in a number of respects:

- The candidate focuses on tasks (e.g. multidisciplinary working, teaching, dealing with difficult patients) rather than skills; the skills which enable him/her to carry out these tasks effectively would be more valuable to mention to the panel (e.g. empathy, active listening).
- The answer discusses the importance of communication rather than the candidate's ability to communicate.
- The candidate does not sell him-/herself (e.g. "okay", "quite").
- The candidate uses language that appears "detached" (e.g. "in my specialty") rather than mentioning said specialty by name, taking ownership of it and make it his/her own personal experience. For instance "Communication is particularly important in restorative dentistry and I have learnt this through my experience in the specialty so far … <continue with examples>".
- Listing English as a language is not relevant. As for the other languages, they do not indicate that the candidate can communicate, but rather that he/she has the told to perhaps relate to patients from certain parts of the world! The link between the languages and how they demonstrate a good ability to communicate should be made more explicit.
- Stating that the skills "obviously can be improved" is a reasonable statement to make; however, mentioned in this manner, it suggests that the candidate is not very good at communication. Instead, the candidate should convey a more positive message by mentioning that he/she is constantly finding opportunities to develop his/her communication skills further (for example, by attending courses such as a recent teaching course). This would create a more positive feeling.

Example of an effective answer

"Throughout my training, I have developed effective communication skills across a wide range of areas. One of my main strengths is my ability to relate to others and empathise with them. During my time in paediatric dentistry, I often dealt with patients who were very apprehensive and required a lot of time, care and attention to gain trust. I found I could engage with patients and their relatives at a level commensurate with their understanding. I can remember quite a few patients who I developed a particular rapport with and was able to inspire confidence in, to ensure they became regular dental attenders and were able to tolerate more complex treatment plans as a result of feeling more comfortable in the clinic.

"As well as this, I feel comfortable expressing my opinions clearly in the different areas of work. I take great care to prepare well to ensure that I don't miss any important points and I take account of what other people want to know and of what they will be doing with the information. For instance, on ward rounds in my time in restorative dentistry, I would focus on salient points and leave aside unimportant details. When discussing a diagnosis or outlining a treatment plan with a patient, I ensure that I take account of their prior knowledge. I can then convey information that I feel will matter to them.

"Over the course of my training so far, I have developed good negotiation and influencing skills. Experience has taught me how everyone in a working environment has their own priorities, pressures and even agendas. I feel that, as I have developed an increased clinical understanding, I have improved my ability to prioritise my patients' needs. This was particularly felt during my time in maxillofacial surgery, where I was often tasked with interfacing with colleagues in roles such as booking emergency theatres and requesting investigations. When dealing with people with conflicting agendas due to competing pressures, I was careful to remain calm, never take things personally and always see things from the perspective of the other person. Constructive discussions would often lead to the best outcomes for patients and sustained productive working relationships between teams.

"In summary, therefore, my key skills of empathy, clarity of expression and constructive inter-professional working are valuable attributes, which will serve me well in a career in restorative dentistry."

8.2 Give an example of a situation where you showed empathy towards a patient

What situations can you describe?

A good example would be a situation where a patient wanted to take a course of action, which you felt was obviously against their best interests. This could be:

- A discharge against medical advice on a maxillofacial surgery rotation
- A refusal of treatment, due to dental anxiety that required patience and a well-developed rapport to overcome
- A failure to comply with post-procedural instructions, e.g. oral hygiene advice, smoking cessation, lifestyle changes
- Compounding psychosocial considerations with limited insight, e.g. atypical facial pain, atypical odontalgia

Whatever example you choose to describe, you must ensure that it is *your* communication skills that made a difference. You must also ensure that you are not seen to coerce the patient into making a decision.

Answering the question

Since this is a question asking for a specific example, you should use the STAR technique (see 5.2).

Example of an effective answer

Situation/Task   "Whilst working in paediatric dentistry, I saw a young boy who had sustained avulsion injuries of both upper central incisors. Whilst the teeth had been stored in milk and he had attended the emergency clinic promptly, he was unwilling to allow anyone to treat him, despite much cajoling from his parents.

Action   "I was able to take him to one of the side clinics, away from the open-plan cubicles in the department, to make sure he felt a little more at ease. I could see from his composure and body language that he wanted to tell me more about what was making him so apprehensive. I felt it was important to let him talk to me in his own time, and I gently asked why he was so apprehensive, providing a calm and reassuring

---

atmosphere. He told me that it was a combination of factors, including previous bad experiences of dental treatment, and the circumstances surrounding his injury, as he had knocked out the teeth whilst skateboarding. A few weeks prior, he had sustained a possible scaphoid fracture doing the same activity and he was very apprehensive about not being allowed to continue.

Result/Reflect   "Once I gained his trust and that of his parents, I was able to complete reimplantation and splinting of the teeth and the first stage of endodontic treatment. I think that by listening actively, preparing the scene and mirroring his pace, as well as talking to his level, I was able to engage with the patient quickly. That groundwork went a long way in securing his trust in both myself and the profession in general. I was even able to convince him to allow me to make him a custom mouth guard and that he would start wearing protective headgear when skateboarding, a compromise he reached with his parents to allow him to continue skateboarding!"

The story describes in some detail how the dentist approached the patient and how he/she made a difference. In this example, there are further opportunities to demonstrate empathy, by discussing how the dentist then handled the patient once he had admitted what the issues were. This would make the answer far too long, however, and it may be best to wait until prompted for more information. Note the reflective paragraph at the end, where the candidate states what he/she did well.

8.3 Describe a time when you had to defend your own beliefs regarding the treatment of a patient

What this question is testing and what the interviewers are looking for?

The interviewers will be looking for a range of skills, including:

- Your ability to listen and take on board criticism without losing your cool
- Your ability to set out your opinions in a constructive manner
- Your ability to influence others in a non-threatening manner

Scenarios you can discuss

Hopefully, this is not a situation that recurs much in your daily working life, so any situation where this has occurred should stand out in your mind. This could be, for example:

- A situation where you made a decision that was queried by one of your peers, or seniors or a nurse, and where you had to defend your views
- A situation where your decision or belief with regard to treatment was queried, either by the patient or one of his/her relatives
- A case review meeting where you were asked to justify your actions

How would you normally seek to convince someone that you are right?

- First, you would ensure that you have all the information to hand, to be able to present a sensible case.

- Secondly, you would present logical arguments to the other person and would wait for their reaction. You would essentially appeal to reason and common ground. Ultimately, both of you want the best outcome for the patient, and it may be a case of seeing each other's perspectives. You may have what are initially perceived to be conflicting interests, but with sufficient discussion, these could be seen to be complementary.

- Be prepared to concede on certain points and compromise when recognising the value of someone else's view, but at the same time make sure you paint a picture of yourself "holding your own" where required, and being the patient's advocate above all else.

- You may wish to appeal to objective evidence, guidelines and evidence-based dentistry (EBD). If evidence in the wider literature or expert opinion supports your perspective, then use this. Remember that senior colleagues in particular may have valid reasons for contradicting guidelines, based on their clinical judgement and experience (they are, after all, "guidelines", and meant to guide rather than order clinicians). They should be prepared to defend themselves when contradicting evidence, however, and these are valuable learning opportunities.

- If your conflict involves a peer, you may recourse to seeking an intermediary, in the form of a senior clinician, if you have reached an impasse following a full and thorough exploration of the options above.

- If none of this works, then there may not be an easy conclusion to the problem. If patients are involved, the complaint procedure or even court action, etc, may need to be invoked. For the purpose of answering this question, you should ensure that you choose an example where you were successful at defending your beliefs, otherwise you will run into trouble, however justified your actions were.

Example of an effective answer

Situation/Task "Whilst working in maxillofacial surgery I saw a patient in the emergency department, who was referred with a fractured mandible. The patient had a depressed level of consciousness, however, which the ED referring doctor had put down to inebriation. However, I suspected a head injury.

Action I spent a couple of minutes assessing the patient and gathering a collateral history from the ambulance crew and a friend who had attended with the patient. I expressed my concerns to the referring doctor, who reiterated that the patient had 'had a skinful' and was likely to be drunk. I felt uncomfortable accepting the referral and pointed out that according to NICE guidelines, a GCS of less than 13/15 warranted a CT head to exclude a co-existing head injury.

The referring doctor continued to be adamant that I was overplaying the situation. As I had failed to achieve a resolution by appealing to reason and objective evidence and guidelines, I contacted my middle grade on call. They spoke to an ED middle grade, and the consensus was that

---

the patient should have a CT, which demonstrated a small depressed frontal fracture with a co-existing pneumocephalus.

Result/Reflect   The patient was referred to neurosurgery, who accepted care, and his mandible was fixed some days later, when safe to transfer care following serial imaging. The ED doctor was very apologetic, but I thought this was a learning experience for all involved. We worked together to produce and deliver a presentation on head injuries to junior staff at ED teaching and at the maxillofacial clinical governance meetings in both departments."

Note the emphasis on communication, listening and being non-judgemental, but at the same time being assertive where required. There is a clear progression through an appeal to common ground and reason, giving the other party room to express his/her opinion and then setting out clearly why you contradict this. This is followed by appealing to objective evidence and allowing the other party a chance to state why they might be deviating from what you and others might regard as best practice (where this exists). Finally, the candidate has resorted to arbitration with a more senior clinician, demonstrating a recognition of hospital/departmental hierarchy and the need to "stick to your guns" and remain an advocate for the best interests of the patient.

Don't be afraid to go into some detail. Detail and facts will help build up your credibility and will bring the example to life. But always make sure that those details are relevant to the question being asked.

You can use the "Result/Reflect" section to explain a little bit more than what happened at the end of the story, by adding a sentence about how it helped you become a better dentist. In this example, it is about building bridges with the referring clinician, in the interests of both personal and institutional learning; and the dissemination of the lessons learnt to a wider audience really puts the finishing touches on the answer.

8.4 Describe a time when your communication skills made a difference to the outcome of patient care

What examples can you use?

The question focuses not just on your communication skills, but on a situation where they actually made a difference to the care of a patient. There are several areas that you can explore, for example:

- Situations where the patient was reluctant to agree to a procedure because, perhaps, they were scared (maybe due to a previous bad experience) or had trouble understanding what it involved
- Situations where the patient had needs that they had not clearly expressed, and which you managed to identify through good communication
- Situations where you communicated well with a range of members of your team, which then led to efficient action towards the care of a patient

Although the question does not specify whether the communication skills should be directed towards the patient or towards the team, we would recommend that you play safe by addressing communication with the patient (i.e. the first two points) rather than with the team, as this is likely to have a greater impact.

Example of an effective answer

Situation/Task   "Whilst working in maxillofacial surgery as a DCT 1, I had a lady present with a submandibular abscess, which needed an urgent admission for incision and drainage. She was very reluctant to come in, and it transpired that her husband, who was disabled as a result of stroke and vascular dementia, was on his own at home and she did not want to leave him by himself.

Action   "I spent some time listening to the patient and trying to show as much empathy as possible so that I could gain her trust. My main aim at that stage was to let her talk so that I could identify how we could compromise with her. I explained to her that we would do our utmost to take care of her husband as well as her, and that one solution would be to involve social services so that her husband would be looked after whilst she was recovering. At first, she was reluctant to involve social services because she felt that her

---

87

husband may be taken away from her. I was able to reassure her that this would not be the case and that her husband would be well looked after.

Result/Reflect   "The patient was happy with this solution and subsequently accepted to be admitted. I felt that I was able to make a real difference, by showing real empathy towards the patient at a difficult time for her, and by looking at the situation as a whole rather than concentrating solely on her physical needs."

This example is effective because the story is easy to follow. The context is set out clearly, as is the action that the candidate took. Note the small amount of clinical information, which is just enough to aid the comprehension of the scenario, without overwhelming the interviewer with unnecessary detail that would distract from the candidate's communication skills.

The final paragraph summarises the main points that the candidate wishes the interviewers to take on board, effectively highlighting how the example given actually answers the question.

8.5 Give an example of a situation where you failed to communicate appropriately

What the interviewers are looking for

This is a question about learning from a communication mistake. The interviewers will be looking for:

- Honesty in acknowledging your mistake (i.e. professionalism and integrity)
- Sensitive and constructive resolution of the problem at the time
- Ability to reflect, learn from your mistake and change your behaviour

When you are asked to incriminate yourself by describing a situation where you failed to act properly, you should avoid fobbing the panel off with comments such as "I can't remember a situation where I did not communicate well because I always do my best to ensure that I provide the best possible care to my patients". This would actually be missing the point of the question.

What examples can you describe?

You can use examples that relate to patients and relatives as well as other team members. This may include:

- Using unnecessary jargon with a patient
- Being too concise in giving instructions to a junior or to a nurse, not appreciating they may not understand you fully
- Assuming a patient is okay with a particular issue and adopting a normal communication approach, when in fact the patient is actually worried and anxious
- Forgetting to give important information to a colleague, which results in a delay in patient care or discharge
- Complaining to a colleague about their behaviour in an abrupt manner, leading to a conflict
- Being insensitive to someone else's point of view in a meeting, leading to a confrontation
- Dealing with a problem via email or a third party, when you would have been better off talking to the person face to face or at least on the phone

The most powerful answers are those based on real and complex problems. If you choose to talk about an insignificant problem, you will not have much to learn from the scenario and will end up with a weak answer. So, be prepared to take risks if you want to score highly.

How did you deal with the problem?

The way in which you handled the matter will obviously have depended on the nature of the problem. For example:

- If your mistake resulted in a patient not adhering to treatment or a colleague doing the wrong thing because they misunderstood you, then you will have needed to make sure that you apologised to the patient or colleague and then explained things again in a better manner.
- If your mistake resulted in a confrontation, then you will have needed to explain how you recognised from their response that you had mishandled the situation, that you apologised and then you corrected the problem by explaining things differently.
- If you were insensitive to someone's point of view at a meeting, you ought to gone and seen them face to face after the event, to apologise and build bridges.

Whatever you did, make sure that you go into enough detail to enable the interviewers to understand that you took the problem seriously and were proactive in resolving the issue.

If the communication problem interfered at any time with patient safety (for example, by delaying treatment because you gave ambiguous instructions), then you must also explain that you took immediate steps to ensure that the patient did not suffer.

Reflect and learn

Once you have described your mistake and how you remedied the situation, reflect on the issues it raises by explaining what you learnt and how you changed your practice thereafter. For example:

> "This scenario showed me how important it is to take the time to check the patient's understanding, even if they seem to have understood, as in this case I would have identified straight away that the patient had not fully grasped the impact of the treatment on their lifestyle. The patient was never at risk, but getting the communication right would have avoided having to call the patient back for further explanation. I now ensure that I systematically check patients' understanding throughout the consultation."

8.6 Tell us about a situation where you had to obtain informed consent from a patient who was in a vulnerable situation

This looks like a question on how to seek consent, so most candidates would rush into describing how they could seek consent (explain advantages and risks, check the person's understanding, etc). However, the question is about much more than that. It specifically relates to a vulnerable patient, and therefore will be testing the sensitivity of your approach and your ability to recognise and adapt to the patient's specific needs.

Identify vulnerable patients you have encountered

This could include:
- Patients who are elderly, of sound mind but easily influenced
- Patients who may be making decisions against their own best interest because of other factors (e.g. fear of becoming a burden on relatives)
- Patients who have just had bad news broken to them
- Patients who have mental health problems
- Patients with learning difficulties, particularly in community / special care dentistry placements

Answering the question

Here again, the STAR system (see 5.2) will help you.

- Start by explaining the context. Who was the patient (ensuring you give enough detail to show how/why they were vulnerable), and what did you need to seek their consent for?

- Detail how you sought consent (explaining things slowly, checking their understanding, drawing diagrams if needed, etc), but throughout your answer, explain how their vulnerability impacted on your actions and how you resolved each problem that this presented you with. For example, simply saying "I explained the procedure in simple terms" is too weak, because this could apply to anyone, not just a vulnerable patient. Instead, you could say something along the lines of "I explained the procedure in simple terms, using a diagram to illustrate my words, but the patient seemed a bit confused about some of the detail and was taking a long time to understand some of the basic information. I therefore asked the nurse and also one of the relatives to explain in their own words what I had described, which helped the patient along. Following our explanation, I asked the patient to tell me in their own words what they thought was going to happen to them. I also made sure that they had an opportunity to ask questions."

- As another example, instead of saying "The patient was crying, so I gave her some leaflets and asked her to come back later", which sounds harsh, you need to explain why you acted in that way and show that you used a sensitive approach that matched the distress of the patient. This could give an answer like "As the patient was crying uncontrollably, I spent some time gently reassuring her that we would do our best for her and asked her if she was okay to continue or wanted to go home. I offered her the opportunity to study some leaflets and come back at a later stage, which she gratefully accepted. She returned three days later", etc.

- Try not to be too technical when explaining how you are seeking consent from the patient, as it is not really the aim of the question (which is how you deal with a vulnerable patient). The only really important consent-seeking aspects for this question are:

  - Explaining the procedure in detail in a clear manner, including pros, cons, alternatives and risks (no need to go into detail in these questions)
  - Checking the understanding of the patient and answering their questions
  - Reassuring the patient that they can change their mind and can take the time to think about their decision

In your example, if you have any doubt about the patient's competence, then make sure that you explain how you sought to check whether they were competent or not (e.g. by calling for help from a consultant or other senior clinician, or involving their general medical practitioner or mental health team).

8.7 What makes you a good team player?

Before you can answer this question, you must understand what being a team player means. Most candidates are able to quote a few of the attributes of a good team player (the most popular one being that a team player understands his role in the team), but they are unable to explain what the attributes mean in practice. This then makes it difficult to provide meaningful examples.

The following sets out and develops the key attributes of a good team player. It will help you crystallise your thoughts and come up with your own ideas and examples:

Qualities of a good team player

Understands their role in the team and how it fits within the whole picture

A good team player understands what is expected of him/her and is able to anticipate and address the needs of other members of the team. He/she must also understand what is expected of others so he/she can work with them effectively. In practice, he/she:

- Is reliable, i.e. delivers quality results in a timely manner and follows through on his/her assignments
- Is consistent, i.e. delivers good quality of work all the time and not just when someone is watching him/her
- Works hard and does his/her fair share of the work; takes responsibility to prioritise and organise his/her work appropriately to deliver results
- Involves others appropriately, e.g. asking for advice or help, referring specific issues to others who have greater knowledge of the problem
- Takes the initiative and works as a problem solver, i.e. does not simply do what they are told, does not blame others, does not avoid getting involved and does not let others deal with problems alone
- Shows commitment to the team; puts the team's success before his/her own pride/success (e.g. if invited to do a non-glamorous task)

Treats others with respect, is supportive and willing to help

A good team player is considerate and courteous towards his/her colleagues. He/she demonstrates understanding and shows appropriate support towards others to help get the job done. An effective team player deals with other people in a professional manner.

In practice, he/she:

- Is consistently approachable (i.e. not just when it suits them)
- Responds to others' requests for help, even if it can be inconvenient
- Takes the initiative to offer help when he/she feels someone needs it
- Allows others to express their opinions and respects them
- Takes into account other people's agendas and feelings
- Goes beyond his/her differences with others and finds ways to work together to get the job done
- Shows diplomacy and tact
- Does not gossip maliciously or attempt to undermine others
- Demonstrates a good sense of humour and knows how to interact with others in a more social context

Is flexible, adaptable and able to compromise

A good team player adapts to ever-changing situations without complaining or resisting. In practice, he/she:

- Can consider different points of view and compromise when needed
- Does not hold rigidly to a point of view, especially when the team needs to move forward to make a decision or get on with things
- Is able to strike a compromise between holding onto his/her own beliefs and convictions, whilst respecting and taking on board others' opinions
- Shows willingness to change working methods to adapt to new circumstances, without complaining, getting stressed or resisting change

Communicating constructively and listening actively

Communication is the lynchpin of any good team, and a good team player encourages and contributes to good communication. In practice, he/she:

- Speaks up and expresses his/her thoughts and ideas clearly, directly, honestly, and with respect for others and for the work of the team
- Proposes ideas that help resolve problems rather than create them
- Absorbs, understands, and considers ideas and points of view from other people without debating and arguing every point
- Avoids interrupting others to force his/her point through
- Is willing to accept and listen to comments or criticisms from others without reacting defensively, even if those comments come from more junior colleagues
- Shares appropriate information with colleagues and keeps them up to date about progress on his/her assignments

Answering the question

It would be tempting to try to work all of the above into a single answer; however, this is likely to sound corny and/or contrived. To answer the question effectively, you must pick three or four of the above skills, which you feel characterise you best, and expand on each, using your past experiences. Spreading three points over two minutes makes it 40 seconds per point, which gives plenty of time for a couple of brief examples.

Example of an effective answer

"One of my key strengths as a team player is definitely my ability to motivate other people when things are not going well and to support them through hard work, and by making myself available to help when required. Over the past few months in my DCT3 job in maxillofacial surgery, I worked with a couple of DCT1s. For many, this was their first experience of maxillofacial surgery and I tried to spend time with them to help them navigate the workload and deal with the stressful nature of the job, as well as supporting them in developing new practical skills such as suturing and looking after the head and neck patients on the ward. I was able to act as a 'senior' SHO, in effect, and took on the role of DCT rep, acting as a go-between for my colleagues and the middle grades / consultants, whilst they were finding their feet.

"As a member of the team, I work very hard to ensure that I do all my jobs on time and with the quality that my colleagues expect of me. I make sure that the handover is kept up to date throughout the shift and ready to seamlessly hand over patient care. I ensure that all investigations are easily accessible to the senior reviewing clinicians on ward rounds. When handing over patients, I try to ensure that any outstanding jobs are done, and where this is impossible, that these are clearly identified for the clinician coming on shift and taking over. I make sure that laboratory work is checked for the major head and neck cases, and that all investigations are done and chased pre-operatively. I always come to theatre lists well prepared, with advanced knowledge of all the patients, their conditions and comorbidities.

"Finally, I have always been very proactive in discussing problems with colleagues so that we can all improve and the team can provide a better service. As an example, I recently identified that many of the day case lists did not match the planned procedures outlined in the notes and letters. I offered to audit the problem and identified a point of weakness in transcribing these accurately, which predisposed to human error. I worked with my registrar and IT to ensure that outcomes from clinics were directly transposed to operating lists and re-audited to demonstrate a reduction in inaccuracies. This ultimately translates

> into improved patient safety, greater efficiency on pre-op ward rounds and a happier, calmer team!"

This example is effective because it focuses on a handful of key points (i.e. it does not simply list 20 attributes of a good team player); each point is clearly backed up with personal experience and presents the candidate as someone who is clearly playing an active role in the team rather than waiting for others to tell him/her what to do, when to do it and how to do it!

8.8 Give an example of a recent situation where you played an important role in a team

This question is asking for a recent example. Typically, this means the last few months. Also, note that the focus of the question is on a situation where teamwork is important, as opposed to a situation where you were a good team player. However, you should not be fooled by this; it is a question about you and your ability to demonstrate good team-playing abilities. You must therefore find an example where you played a key role.

Examples that you can use

Identify a situation in your recent past where you have had the opportunity to demonstrate a range of team-playing skills set out in the previous question. This could be a situation where you:

- Participated in the organisation of an event or project such as organising a seminar, regular teaching sessions, regional British Dental Association (BDA) events, oral cancer-screening days, etc.

- Had to deal with a complex patient, where team playing was important. In order to make the answer interesting, you would need to find an example where you had to deal with a multidisciplinary team, e.g. a hypodontia patient. You could then explain how you participated in the debate about the treatment plan.

- Developed a treatment plan that engaged the help of dental care professionals (DCPs), e.g. hygienist, orthodontic therapist, dental nursing staff, dental technicians. Critically, you should have been responsible for the overarching treatment plan and coordinating input.

- Had to deal with an emergency by using the staff resources available, whilst maintaining constant communication with your seniors so that they could have an input into the process and would be fully briefed by the time they arrived. Note that, in order to highlight as many skills as possible, you would need to ensure that the situation was complex enough to show how your role was key to the success of the team, e.g. making a timely referral to hospital for a cervicofacial infection requiring admission; dealing with a medical emergency in the clinic.

Example of an ineffective answer

"I work every day as part of a team, dealing with my dental nursing staff and members of the dental team. I am aware of my limitations and seek help when necessary, and I communicate with everyone in the team. I am willing to help and motivate others."

This answer is too vague and general. In fact, it does little more than summarise the job description. Also, it does not actually answer the question, which is asking for *an example* of a recent situation, i.e. a specific scenario in which you were involved.

Another example of an ineffective answer

"I saw a patient in an oral medicine clinic, who had a suspicious ulcer on the tongue but refused a biopsy. I talked to the nurse and the consultant, and eventually the patient relented and agreed to have the biopsy performed. The diagnosis proved to be an oral squamous cell carcinoma, and the patient went on to be referred to a local maxillofacial department for definitive treatment."

This answer follows the STAR structure, which is a plus point. It starts well, by explaining the context that leads to the team action being started. However, the "Action" section contains very little information:

- Why did the candidate talk to the dental nurse or the consultant? Probably because the consultant is responsible for the patient and had to be informed. As for the nurse, it might have been because she had a good rapport with the patient or could help put the patient at ease. This needs to be explained.

- Did the candidate do anything else that would have shown him/her to be a good team player, for example, taking the initiative to contact social services, or asking the patient if the relatives could be involved?

The answer basically needs more details about what was done and why it was done. In addition, the "Result" section is partially addressing the wrong point. As well as highlighting that the problem was satisfactorily resolved, it should emphasise that this was the result of teamwork.

Example of an effective answer

"During my maxillofacial DCT1 year, I was called to the resuscitation area of the emergency department to see a patient with suspected Ludwig's angina. I recognised the potential severity of this situation at the outset, so informed my registrar of where I was going, prior to setting off from the clinic.

"Upon arrival, it was apparent to me that the patient had a very distended neck bilaterally and was struggling to breathe. I made sure that all the emergency measures were in place, such as oxygen and intravenous access, and contacted the on-call anaesthetist to come and assess the patient's airway and get him ready for theatres. I contacted my registrar to alert them about the situation and then contacted the theatre coordinator to ensure a second emergency theatre was opened up.

"Whilst awaiting the arrival of the anaesthetist, I made sure I got all the investigations ready, and worked in conjunction with the nurse in the resuscitation bay, to ensure the patient was kept safe and that senior ED clinicians were aware of his presence and my potential need for help.

"The patient was taken to theatre that night for incision and drainage of the submandibular spaces and removal of a lower third molar and ended up spending the night intubated on the intensive care unit. Subsequently, however, he made a full recovery. I recognised the importance of knowing my limitations and keeping everyone in the loop in an evolving situation. Whilst I had to ask for a lot of help, I was effectively the lynchpin in ensuring the patient got the care he needed."

The answer works well on a number of levels:

- The candidate recognises his/her limitations.
- He/she informs his/her seniors and keeps them up to date about developments.
- He/she informs colleagues about developments that are relevant to them and engages their help early on in the situation (e.g. anaesthetist).
- He/she uses other team members to help out based on their skill levels.
- Finally, the candidate gets things done (stabilising the patient, preparing theatres, etc).

Whilst the candidate had some limitations, by virtue of their junior level of training, there was a clear recognition of the value of contribution to patient care as a "lynchpin". Remember not only to highlight the outcome, but also what you did to make this possible and your role. Without this element of reflection, the answer will achieve a low score.

8.9 Give an example of a situation where you failed to act as a good team player

Like all negative questions asking you to incriminate yourself, you must make sure that you choose an example that helps you sell your potential. The interviewers will be testing:

- Your self-awareness, i.e. your ability to recognise your faults, reflect on situations and determine what you did wrong

- Your ability to learn from your bad experiences and change your behaviour accordingly

Examples that you can discuss

Essentially, you need to consider the qualities of a good team player (see 8.7) and identify whether you have examples of situations where you acted against any of these. This could include a situation where:

- You failed to complete a task that you were entrusted to do and, when you realised that you would struggle to complete it, you did not inform the person who had asked you to do it.

- You did complete the task or project that you were entrusted to run, but you were so busy that you did not give it your full attention and the quality of your work suffered, i.e. you became complacent.

- You had some important personal issues to resolve and thought it would be okay to leave a little early. You chose not to let anyone know and, unfortunately, someone actually needed your help.

- You attended a meeting where you had a "heated debate" with someone because you focused a bit too much on trying to impose your point of view rather than listening to what they had to say.

- One of your colleagues was struggling or needed some help, but you felt it was someone else's job to do it.

- You were uncomfortable in changing your approach to a particular problem, despite receiving advice from colleagues because you felt you were right (but ended up being wrong).

- Someone suggested a change in working practices, but you resisted the change because you couldn't see the point. You failed to consider the new approach and ended up causing friction.

- You felt that something was not quite right in the way some aspects of patient care or departmental life were organised and decided to let it go because you felt your input would not make much difference (or that you were about to rotate anyway).

- You had information that would make a difference to a particular issue but did not feel confident raising it (though this may be dangerous to mention because the interviewers may feel that you would be reluctant to report a problem colleague, for example).

- You carried out a task by yourself instead of involving other appropriate people, because you felt it would be easier or quicker to get on with it. Your colleagues then became upset (once again, consider this option carefully, as your interviewers may view you as tending to work beyond your limitations).

Structuring your answer

To give your answer the maximum impact, you must ensure that the emphasis is on the learning points rather than on your unsatisfactory actions. The following approach would be successful in achieving this:

Situation/Task	Describe the situation, your behaviour and the negative impact that it had (e.g. someone became upset). State clearly why you feel you did not demonstrate appropriate team-playing behaviour.
Action	Explain how you resolved the problem at the time (e.g. did you have to work harder to compensate for your failure or attempt to build bridges with colleagues you had upset?)
Result/Reflect	How did the story finish? What did you learn from the situation and how do you feel it has altered your behaviour? This is the most crucial part of the answer. Make sure that there is a strong learning point and, if you can (and if you've got time), briefly describe another situation that demonstrates that you have now altered your behaviour.

8.10 Do you work better on your own or as part of a team?

This question is often misunderstood and sees candidates rushing to reassure the interviewers that, since they are good team players, they work better as part of a team. The answer is slightly more complex and requires you to demonstrate that, although you are, of course, a good team player, you can also work independently (though still within the remit of a team), i.e. that you are not someone who requires constant support to get on with their work.

One way to structure the answer is to have two sections: one where you describe how you can work independently, followed by a section on how you can also work as part of a team. Alternatively, you can structure your answer around different types of work that you do, showing how you can be independent and also a team player.

Example of an effective answer

"The answer to this question is that I can work well, both as part of a team and independently, depending on what the situation calls for. When I arrive in the morning for the orthodontic clinic, I ensure that the clinic list is reviewed, study models are available and ready, treatment plans are made prior to arrival as far as possible, radiographs are all available for review, and any inter-disciplinary opinions, e.g. surgical review / restorative dentistry review, are to hand. Although I take full ownership of this task, it is a clearly defined role and often requires me to use my own initiative; by fulfilling this job well, I function as a team player at the same time. Indeed, I need to anticipate what information my colleagues are likely to need when making management decisions; I also often need to liaise with other departments when information is missing, which requires good communication and, sometimes, diplomacy.

"When I undertake my audit projects, a lot of the work required consists of data collection and analysis. I like to take full responsibility for all of this and make sure that I deliver what is required, by working independently. However, I also involve my senior colleagues when I need to discuss a particular issue relating to the project; and if one of my junior colleagues is keen to get involved, I will make sure that they can take part in the project too. I think that part of being a good team player is also to be able to undertake roles and work independently, delivering what the team requires of you, whilst ensuring that you maintain constant communication. I feel that it is something that I am particularly good at, and my colleagues' feedback is that I am a proactive and entrepreneurial individual who is, at the same time, attentive to others' needs and also a strong communicator."

8.11   What makes you a good leader?

What is leadership?

Leadership can be described in three words: **Change – People – Results**

Initiating and implementing change
A leader is someone who has a vision of how departments or teams should develop or change and is able to drive that change. He/she is able to question conventional wisdom and current practice, to encourage others to develop their own ideas and to implement new protocols, guidelines or new ways of working. This involves building relationships with others, not just within your own environment, but also with others outside, to ensure greater collaboration and achieve common goals. Leadership is also about identifying and understanding the impact of internal and external politics and acting accordingly. That involves negotiating and influencing others, building consensus and gaining cooperation from others, to ensure that the right information is obtained and that common objectives are achieved.

Developing people (and creating a positive environment)
A leader takes people with him/her towards the objectives that he/she has set and makes sure that he/she creates an environment in which people can develop, work together and cooperate, and where there are good mechanisms in place to resolve conflicts constructively.

Delivering results
This is the ability to meet set goals and expectations. This includes an ability to make decisions that lead to tangible results, by applying knowledge, analysing problems and calculating risks. Delivering results is the aspect of leadership to which you are most usually exposed as a trainee, and is the closest to management. Essentially, it is about organising a team, planning and delegating, and getting things done.

You don't have to be a clinical director to be a leader!

Leadership is a real skill that anyone can demonstrate. You don't have to be a consultant or a chief executive to exercise leadership. We are often struck by the number of people who ask us at our courses: "How do they expect us to demonstrate leadership when we are only trainees?" In truth, you probably started demonstrating leadership very early in your career, and even before. For example, anyone who has had to deal with a busy on-call or with multiple emergencies on their own, or with limited resources, would be demonstrating leadership – even leading a ward round and the organisation surrounding that may be an example. This section should help you clarify your thoughts and will prompt you to think about your own examples.

Qualities of a leader

From the description of leadership set out above, you can see that the following list constitutes the requirements of a good leader:

Approachable	Encouraging	Integrity
Assertive	Fair	Open-minded
Clear communicator	Fast learner	Organised
Consistent	Flexible	Patient
Constructive	Good listener	Resilient
Creative	Honest	Supportive
Decisive	Innovative	Tenacious
Diplomatic		

Answering the question

What makes you a good leader will be a mixture of the responsibilities that you take and your personal qualities, both of which you can derive from the issues above. Leadership is a vast topic, and you should ensure that you focus on three or four areas or skills that you feel represent you and your experience best; attempting to discuss everything will either result in a superficial or a very long answer.

Example of an effective answer

"One of my strengths as a leader is that I take ownership of a task, a project or a problem when it is given to me. I also involve the other members of my team, to ensure that we work well together towards completing that project. For example, in the busy practice where I spent my dental foundation training, I would often have to prioritise emergency patients, whilst still dealing with the workload of the planned patients for the day. As a leader in these stressful situations, I feel that I am very good at keeping the dental team together, by maintaining good communication with everyone, delegating appropriately to dental care professionals and maintaining meticulous organisation, to manage what was at times a seemingly insurmountable workload.

"As a leader, I am very supportive and encouraging towards my colleagues. I try my absolute best to ensure that I encourage others in the team to consolidate their skills and experience, as well as developing new aspects of their practice. In the dental practice where I worked for some time as an associate, I introduced a sedation service and encouraged some of the nursing staff to attend the Society for the Advancement of Anaesthesia in Dentistry course. Two of the nurses became SAAD accredited assistants, and we ran regular updates within the practice to ensure our skills were up to date. I also organised regular workshops for the MFGDP examinations and journal clubs, to ensure that we were cohesive as a team in our approach to grow together in providing the best possible evidence-based care to our patients.

"Finally, I have a good ability to engage with people, even when conflicts develop. For example, since moving back into dental hospital jobs, I have had to deal with referring GDPs who insist that a patient who could seemingly be managed in the community be accepted for treatment in the dental hospital. In these situations I have always tried my best to keep calm, see the perspective of others and make appropriate concessions, but firmly explain my point of view when this is in the patients' best interests (and in the best interests of resource management). Ultimately, my aim is always to find a constructive way of resolving any problem that ensures the optimal care for the patients, learning for all involved and long-lasting working relationships, and I regularly receive feedback in my multi-source feedbacks attesting to this attitude in my approach to leadership."

This answer is effective because:

- It has three points, which are clearly signposted at the start of each paragraph and demonstrate wide-ranging experience, with examples.

- Each point is expanded just enough to show the extent of the candidate's experience.

- The candidate reflects on his/her skills by demonstrating their impact on others. Bringing feedback into the answer (last paragraph) helps to introduce some objectivity into the answer.

- The candidate uses positive language, and also appears realistic, by presenting the image of someone who, despite being confident, can also involve others and ask for assistance.

8.12 Give an example of a situation where you showed leadership

Choosing the best example

For this question, you should familiarise yourself with the role and qualities of a leader discussed in the previous questions and try to determine which examples would enable you to best present your leadership abilities.

Initiating and implementing change

- Any situation where you identified a problem in the workplace and took the initiative to implement a solution. Maybe you spotted some inefficiency or lack of compliance, did an audit to identify the extent of the problem and then tried to encourage your team to change its practice. Perhaps you identified some training issues and took it upon yourself to liaise with other key team members to change some aspects of training.

- Situations where you held positions of responsibility and were instrumental in making decisions that impacted on other people (for example, if you were on the board of a student committee at dental school).

Developing people and creating a positive environment

- Any team environment / meeting where you have encouraged and managed differences of opinions (e.g. clinics, MDT meetings)

- Situations where you have dealt with a conflict with colleagues in a constructive manner (e.g. an underperforming colleague)

- Projects or tasks where you played a key role in encouraging and supporting juniors or other colleagues, developing their skills and abilities, by providing feedback and encouragement, and providing them with opportunities to become involved in interesting or stretching projects (e.g. audit, teaching or other projects)

- Situations where you sought to encourage a positive team spirit. This could be either through encouragement whilst dealing with a difficult work situation, or even outside of work (e.g. by organising team events such as quizzes or sports tournaments)

Delivering results

- Competently managing a difficult case, with little senior help
- Dealing with multiple emergencies in an under-resourced environment
- Dealing with a difficult patient or a complaint
- Being confronted with a sensitive problem with no immediate help (e.g. child protection issue or any other challenging situation)
- Facing tight deadlines to complete a complex project (e.g. publication for which you need advice from a senior who couldn't care less)
- Negotiating referral of a patient to an acute hospital where the receiving clinician refuses to accept
- Requesting a scan from radiology, who refused to perform it
- Situation where a GP or GDP requested something unreasonable and you needed to "educate" him/her about your position
- Any negotiating situation outside of dentistry, for example if you were in charge of organising an event, or were part of a committee, and had to influence other people to help you with your project, when they were reluctant to engage

Delivering the answer

Delivering the answer should be done using the STAR approach, (see 5.2), ensuring that you use the story as a backdrop to your leadership skills (the whole point of the question is to give you an opportunity to show off your leadership skills, not just the story itself).

Example of an effective answer

Situation/task
"A few months ago, an elderly lady was admitted to the hospital where I was based, as the maxillofacial DCT, with a submandibular abscess from a carious lower right first molar. She was maintaining her airway and speaking in full sentences, so the decision was taken to delay her surgery until the following morning. Overnight, however, she began to deteriorate.

Action
I made sure that I informed the on-call SpR so that she could advise and be aware of the situation. I made sure that I informed theatres of an impending deterioration in the patient's condition and asked for the on-call anaesthetist to come and assess her airway at the earliest opportunity. In the meantime, I placed a nasopharyngeal airway and asked the nursing staff to

---

	start high-flow oxygen through a non-rebreathe mask, whilst I established intravenous access and gave the patient a dose of antibiotics.
Results	The family arrived, and I was able to convey to them our concerns regarding the patient and the need to take her to theatre overnight. When the SpR arrived, theatres were ready to receive the patient; the SpR was aware of the full extent of the situation, with all salient investigations to hand, and the anaesthetist prepared for a fibreoptic awake intubation.
Reflection	This was a medical emergency. I placed the patient's care and treatment as the highest priority. I was working with a good team and with good planning, delegation and appropriate communication; everyone understood their role and completed it well. By carefully coordinating the actions of a wide range of colleagues, I was able to make sure the team delivered efficient and safe care to the patient and her family."

This example is effective because it describes in detail the candidate's actions, with sufficient clinical information and clear reflection at the end of the answer.

8.13 What is the difference between management and leadership?

In a nutshell, leadership is setting a new direction or vision for a group, and developing colleagues in a team. Management is about controlling or directing people/resources in a group, according to principles or values that have already been established.

The differences between leadership and management can be illustrated by considering what happens when you have one without the other.

Leadership without management ... sets a direction or vision that others follow, without considering too much how the new direction is going to be achieved. Other people then have to work hard in the trail that is left behind, picking up the pieces and making it work. In dentistry, this could be a consultant who asks trainees or nurses to manage a patient in a certain way, without making sure that it is realistic, or without understanding the hurdles that could be met on the way.

Management without leadership ... controls resources to maintain the status quo or ensure things happen according to already-established plans. For example, a referee manages a sports game, but does not usually provide "leadership" because there is no new change, no new direction – the referee is controlling resources to ensure that the laws of the game are followed and status quo is maintained. In dentistry, this would be a dentist who ensures that protocols and guidelines are followed, without questioning, when necessary, whether they are actually applicable or relevant. It would also be a dentist who gets things done but does not worry about finding opportunities to train and develop his/her trainees.

Leadership combined with management ... does both – it sets a new direction *and* manages the resources to achieve it, for example a newly elected prime minister.

8.14 Give an example of a situation where a new and different approach to a patient of yours proved beneficial

What is this question about?

Essentially, the question is asking you to describe a situation where your first approach was unsuccessful, and where you then changed your strategy of approach to achieve your objective. This could include situations where:

- A patient was reluctant to go ahead with one of your recommendations and where you had to take a different approach in your communication to ensure that they got the message.

- The first approach that you used with a patient revealed some hidden issues, which then prompted you to choose a different approach. For example, you may have adopted a "standard" approach to the problem but then gained information from the patient that indicated there were deeper psychological issues at stake, which needed to be resolved as part of the same process.

This question is testing three skills:

- Your ability to think laterally about a difficult situation, using your knowledge of the patient/situation and the resources available to you in order to find a solution that will drive you towards a successful outcome (note that this could include involving other people such as relatives, other healthcare professionals, etc, in which case you may be able to include an element of teamwork in your answer)

- Your communication skills in relation to the patient

- The manner in which you are able to build and maintain a rapport with the patient to achieve your desired objective, whilst not compromising your integrity, but preserving respect for the patient's values and choices

Delivering the answer

This is a question asking for a specific example, so you should use the STAR structure (see 5.2), ensuring that you do not provide too much clinical information, that you describe clearly the steps that you took to achieve the desired result, and that you mention the outcome. If appropriate, you should reflect on the situation to highlight what you did well.

Example of an ineffective answer

"During my DFT year, an 18-year-old patient came to my practice with dental neglect and poor oral hygiene. He had a very poor track record of attendance at the practice. Despite my best efforts to explain the situation to the patient and encourage him to attend, he was not listening attentively and was being uncooperative. I felt a stronger approach would be required to spur the patient into action. I told him that, unless he took on board advice regarding oral hygiene and smoking cessation, as well as becoming a regular dental attender, the long-term result would likely be that many of his teeth would become unrestorable and require extraction, possibly even a full dental clearance."

The above answer has many good points: it deals with a specific example, the situation is fairly clear, and the clinical information is reduced to the bare minimum. However, it seems a little harsh. The candidate is saying "He wouldn't listen, so I scared him to make him comply". This needs to be softened. In particular, he/she should spend more time demonstrating how he/she approached the patient in the first place, in order to demonstrate why the second approach was then necessary.

Also, the candidate has missed out the "Result" part of the answer. This makes it look very odd and even scary, to a point. You simply don't feel that there was a rapport between the patient and the candidate, or any attempt by the candidate to try his/her very best before escalating his/her approach. The answer should therefore focus more around the communication aspect and how he/she interacted with the patient, rather than just about what the candidate felt and what he/she said.

Example of an effective answer

Situation/Task   "During my DFT year, an 18-year-old patient came to my practice with widespread dental caries and poor oral hygiene. He had a very poor track record of attendance at the practice. When I enquired about the reasons for his non-attendance, the patient mentioned that he was very apprehensive about dental visits, as he had had some very negative experiences in childhood. He also stated that he often didn't want to make time to attend as he regarded this as the last in his list of priorities unless he had toothache, in which case he attended as an emergency.

Action   "My first approach to the patient's reaction was to listen to him carefully and then explain that I understood his dilemma, emphasising the solutions we could find. I took him through the features of periodontal disease and caries and explained that there were ways in which both disease processes could be controlled. In view of his worries, I reassured him that we could start with simple treatments and progressively introduce more complex treatments as he felt more comfortable. We discussed options for having the more involved treatment, with intravenous sedation as an adjunct, and I also ensured that he was given smoking cessation advice and written information about strategies to quit smoking, as well as an appointment with the practice hygienist. In addition, given his record of poor compliance and attendance, and after discussing my proposed approach with my trainer, I explained to the patient that, unless he took on board advice regarding oral hygiene and smoking cessation, as well as becoming a regular dental attender, the long-term result would likely be that many of his teeth would become unrestorable and require extraction. I reassured him that we would work together as a team to make sure that we did everything possible to restore and maintain his dental health.

Result/Reflect "This resulted in a drastic change in the patient's attitude, and he very quickly agreed to my management plan. A few months later, the patient thanked me for my empathic but assertive approach, as he felt I had turned his behaviour around and ensured that he had a healthy and well-maintained dentition."

This answer is more balanced: showing empathy, discussing with the trainer and then adapting the style of communication to the situation and the patient's reaction, whilst being given against a backdrop of all the pharmacological and non-pharmacological options for managing patient anxiety that impacted on the patient's compliance and attendance record.

It would be easy to mishandle the question by taking a very clinical perspective; this would lead you straight to disaster. There is no harm in presenting clinical information, but only to the extent that it helps towards the story. In the example above, it was necessary to demonstrate the gravity of the patient's condition and the extent to which the patient was "scared" into concordance. Finally, beware of words that may sound harsher than you mean them to be. For example, "I told" is very direct, whilst "I explained" is softer.

8.15 Describe a time when you were unsure whether what you were being told represented the patient's true thoughts or feelings

What type of examples can you discuss?

The question does not clarify whether it is the patient who is not telling you their true thoughts, or whether it is a relative who is telling you something that does not match the patient's thoughts or feelings.

If it is the patient, then it may be because they are frightened of what will happen to them if they reveal their thoughts or feelings. This may be a patient who is scared about their own health problems or diagnosis; a patient who hides part of their history to avoid confronting the reality of their illness; or an elderly patient who is keen to have their health problems resolved but is not keen to be taken into care, who might also be worried about becoming a burden on their relatives.

If it is a relative, it may be that they are trying to forcibly influence the patient into a position that suits them rather than the patient, particularly in the case of paediatric patients or those who lack capacity. More often, it is relatives or carers who feel they have little or no control over their family's healthcare. They often want to help and, whilst the strong expression of their views may be well intentioned, it is often misplaced or misguided.

Which skills are being tested?

The interviewers will be testing:

- Your listening skills, with a particular interest in how you recognised that there was a problem – recognising the issue will come from your own judgement of the situation, based maybe on inconsistencies in the story that you are getting from the patient, their body language, the way they express themselves (for example, by being vague), etc. Ultimately, this will come from your ability to listen to the patient.

- Your empathy, sensitivity and diplomacy. Dealing with the issue is complex and requires you to gain the patient's confidence in order to put them back on the right track. This requires diplomacy and sensitivity.

- Teamwork. You may need to involve:
    - A dental nurse
    - Another healthcare professional, if in a hospital setting
    - Another dental care professional

- The patient's GP
- The patient's regular general dental practitioner
- Your seniors

If you judge that the relatives are causing the problem (for example, by forcing the patient to adopt a particular attitude against his/her will), you may have to use other tools to minimise their possible negative influence on the patient. This could include involving seniors, behaving in an assertive but sensitive manner, spending time with the relatives (after all, there may be a valid reason or fear behind their behaviour), etc.

Example of an ineffective answer

"During my time in oral and maxillofacial surgery, one of the trauma patients wanted to self-discharge because she felt her dog would be in danger if she did not get back home as soon as possible. I suggested that she called a relative so that they could look after the animal, but she was adamant that she needed to do it herself. This prompted me to think that there was more to her story and, after much discussion, I concluded that she was worried about the anaesthesia. In order to resolve the situation, I arranged for the patient to have a second discussion with the anaesthetist and also arranged for a nurse to sit in with her. After the discussion, the patient was happy and went through with the operation."

This answer is not "bad". It has a number of positive aspects:
- It deals with a specific situation.
- The introduction is descriptive, and effective in setting out the situation.
- It addresses the right type of issue.

On the negative side, it describes what the dentist did, but not really why he/she thought or acted like this. In other words, the answer needs more depth and needs to highlight how the dentist used his/her skills to resolve the situation.

Look at the following statement: "This prompted me to think that there was more to her story and, after much discussion, I concluded that she was worried about the anaesthesia." Essentially, it looks as if the candidate has jumped to a conclusion without really explaining how it came about. The whole process has been summarised by "after much discussion". The candidate would need to go into more detail about that conversation and discuss how they spent time with the patient, discussing the situation and their fears, eventually picking up on parts of the conversation that seemed to indicate that she was afraid of having an anaesthetic.

The candidate also needs to emphasise how they used listening skills and empathy to gain the patient's trust and confidence. Perhaps they also asked a nurse to have a conversation with the patient instead, because they felt the nurse had a better rapport with the patient and that the patient would open up more to them.

Example of an effective answer

Situation/Task   "One of my patients wanted to self-discharge because she felt that her dog would be in danger if she did not get back home as soon as possible. I suggested that she called a relative so that they could look after the animal, but she was adamant that she needed to do it herself. This prompted me to think that there was more to her story and that, maybe, she feared the operation she was due to have the next day.

Action   "During a quiet period, I asked a nurse to make sure that I would not be disturbed. I sat down with the patient and asked her gently to tell me about her dog. I listened patiently to her, showing an interest in her story and occasionally asking questions. As the patient opened up to me, I felt more comfortable about introducing the subject of her own health and the operation. I could feel that she wanted to express her fears but that she was reluctant to admit to the problem, perhaps because she did not want to appear foolish. I gently explained what the operation entailed and reassured her about the anaesthesia. In order to avoid giving the patient the impression that I was pressurising her, I asked the nurse to spend some time with her. To reassure the patient further, I arranged a meeting with the anaesthetist and arranged for the relatives to discuss the care of the dog with the patient.

Result/Reflect   "After a few hours of concerted teamwork and sensitive communication, the patient agreed to remain in hospital, and the surgery went ahead as scheduled, with a successful outcome. I feel that I played an important role in achieving a good outcome for the patient, despite her initial reluctance to open up, not only by recognising some of her unspoken needs, but also by giving her the time and attention that she needed to open up, without coercing her."

This example combines teamwork and communication skills in a relatively detailed manner. To have an impact, you must make sure that your answers are as personal as they can be, by drawing on the relevant detail of the experience that you have accumulated over the years. The above example also shows you how you can transform an "okay" answer into a much more precise answer, simply by expanding on one or two ideas that you raised, highlighting how you used your skills in practice to achieve the desired result.

8.16 Describe a situation when you had to use creative thinking to solve a problem at work

What is creative thinking?

Many candidates who are confronted with this question struggle to find appropriate examples, not because they are short of experience but simply because they struggle with the wording of the question, and particularly the meaning of the term "creative thinking".

If you struggle with some words in the question, it is of course perfectly acceptable to ask the interviewers for clarification so that you have a chance to present the best possible answer, though of course it may cost you a small amount of marks. However, losing a few marks for seeking clarification is far better than scoring none for going down completely the wrong path.

"Creative thinking" refers to the fact that you have used your imagination and initiative to resolve a problem. In the marking schedule, the interviewers would be looking for the following indicators:

- Capacity to use logic and lateral thinking to solve problems and make decisions
- Capacity to think beyond the obvious, with an analytical and flexible mind
- Capacity to bring a range of approaches to problem solving
- Demonstration of effective judgement and decision-making skills

Examples you can discuss

The question relates to a situation with which you were unfamiliar, and for which you had to use your brain power to develop a sensible and effective solution. This may include situations where:

- You had to deal with a patient who presented with a condition that you were unfamiliar with.

- Your senior asked you to organise something that you had never organised before (educational meeting, audit project, rota, etc).

- You had to deal with several tasks at the same time, which looked completely impossible to you at the time (for example, routine work and several emergencies all at the same time).

- You have a patient who looks like he has a particular condition, but something tells you that there is more to it than meets the eye. Your creative thinking leads you to do some reading in textbooks and on the Internet, before having a chat with your senior. You also feel that another dentist from a different department can help, so you contact them and arrange a discussion on the patient's condition, to find a solution to your problem.

- You work in a dental hospital where the timetable seems to result in a disparity in or lack of training opportunities in certain areas. You come up with a solution of your own, discuss it with your colleagues and then arrange a meeting with a consultant to discuss the problems caused by the current system and to offer your own ideas. As a result, your proposal is implemented.

- You are running a clinic where you constantly have the same problem with patients. For example, they need to take simple information away with them after the clinic, but that information often gets scribbled on a piece of paper, which they lose. You take the initiative to produce a proforma slip, which other clinicians can complete quickly by ticking the right boxes, and which patients are less likely to ignore.

- You have discovered that members of your team often forget to consider certain points in their history taking, which slows down patient management and may lead to errors. You know that the current system has been implemented by a consultant who thinks that it works well, and you need to convince everyone that the system needs to be changed. Your creative thinking leads you to use diplomacy and tact to highlight the issue and to offer a counter-solution, without upsetting the consultant in question.

- You are on call in oral and maxillofacial surgery as a DCT, facing a difficult case, and none of your seniors are available for help. You can then describe the research you did to find a solution and how you used other resources available (nurses' advice, other juniors/seniors from other wards) to solve your problem.

Delivering the answer

As this is a question asking for an example, you will need to use the STAR approach used in such previous questions (see 5.2). You should conclude on a personal note, for example by mentioning how the situation helped you gain confidence in your own abilities to handle complex scenarios, or how it made you realise how important it was to use the resources available to you and to work as a team.

Example of an effective answer

Situation/Task   "In the dental hospital where I was based for dental core training, a lot of patients were seen in various departments with temporomandibular joint disorders. There was quite a lot of inconsistency in the information that was recorded during the history and examination, and in the decision-making surrounding imaging, initial treatment and specialist referral.

Action   "I suggested to my consultant that we should consider having a proforma to enable salient history points as well as examination findings to be recorded. This would standardise the information recorded, to ensure that it was comparable, that nothing was missed and that everybody was singing from the same hymn sheet. It would also serve as a template for specialist referrals.

Result/Reflect   "My suggestion was subsequently approved and implemented within clinics, in areas as diverse as oral medicine, oral surgery and paediatric dentistry. This was an issue that had often been talked about amongst my colleagues but never addressed. Most people felt that it would be too much hard work to convince anyone to effect a change, particularly since all the consultants never seemed to have any time to discuss such matters. However, by anticipating the information that they would need to make a decision, gathering all the information, and presenting a case in a simple and concise format, I was able to streamline consultations with an often challenging patient cohort. The unexpected effect was a simultaneous reduction in consultation times but improvement in satisfaction scores by patients, following an audit undertaken by myself and my colleagues. This was in turn presented at the British Association of Oral Surgeons annual meeting, and other dental hospitals have expressed an interest in introducing their own TMJ history-taking proforma."

This answer is effective because the issue is clearly set out and well explained. The "Action" section is not confined to what the candidate did, but explains why he/she took such steps, and demonstrates that the clinician anticipates the impact of his/her actions on others. This reflects a good level of influencing skills (i.e. the ability to get things done without coercing anyone), which would score highly.

The example above is a clinical example; however, it would be perfectly acceptable to discuss a non-clinical scenario, using the same principles. If you have any doubt as to whether the interviewers require a clinical scenario or not, ask them to clarify the wording of the question.

8.17 Tell us about a mistake that you have made

What the question is testing

This question is testing your ability to recognise that you make mistakes, to take responsibility for your mistakes, to sort them out, to reflect on your experience, to modify your behaviour accordingly and to ensure that others benefit from your experience too.

Many candidates are reluctant to discuss their mistakes because they feel that it will present them as bad clinicians. However, with this question, the interviewers are trying to establish that you are safe in a realistic context; as far as you are concerned, this means demonstrating that when mistakes happen, you can deal with them appropriately (and not that you never make mistakes – if you said that, you would score zero).

Structuring an answer

You will need to follow the STAR structure (see 5.2). For this question, this will mean bringing the following items into your answer, all of which would be reflected in the marking scheme:

Example of an effective answer

Situation/Task   Describe the scenario (keeping the clinical information to the strict minimum necessary to the comprehension of the story). Explain what the mistake was and its impact (i.e. how did that affect the patient, if at all).

Action   Explain the clinical steps that you followed to resolve the problem and make sure that the patient was safe. Describe which other members of the team you involved and why you needed to involve them. Describe how you communicated with the patient or relatives about the mistake made (this is often neglected by most candidates, thus costing them valuable marks).

Result/Reflect   Reflect on the scenario and explain what you have learnt from it. Explain how it changed your practice, perhaps giving a quick example of a different situation where you acted differently. Explain how you ensured that others

---

> learnt from it (for example, by raising the problem at a team meeting / sending an email to others). If you completed a critical incident form, don't forget to mention it.

Which mistakes can you mention?

A good answer will discuss a mistake that is:

- Personal, i.e. your mistake and not that of another colleague. If you talk about someone else's mistake, you will miss the opportunity to demonstrate your own integrity.

- Interesting, i.e. which has some element of drama. If the mistake is boring to describe, it is likely to score low. Similarly, if you choose a mistake that is fairly common, then you are less likely to impress, unless the consequences were significant enough to make the whole answer interesting.

- Safe. You don't want to appear completely incompetent. "Safe" does not mean that no harm was caused to the patient, but that, if there was harm or risk of serious harm, you identified it quickly and took immediate steps to resolve the problem. AVOID NEVER EVENTS, e.g. wrong site extractions. Examples that are safe would include any near misses, any situation where the patient was inconvenienced or non-emergency care was delayed, or even any situation where the patient was placed at risk but you recognised it before much harm could be caused, e.g. wrong side inferior dental blocks (downgraded from a never event in 2019, following lobbying from the BDA). Everyone on your panel will know what being a dentist is like. There is no point pretending that you are perfect.

- Good learning ground. Half the marks will relate to the learning points that you drew from the experience and how you changed your practice. If your example is too safe, you are unlikely to have any interesting learning points and will end up scoring a low mark. For this reason, you want to avoid any mistakes that are not yours; any mistakes that are caused by a system failure; and any mistakes that are in fact recognised complications, since it is only with hindsight that you could say that something could have been done differently.

For all clinical mistakes, it is important to include the fact that you completed an incident form. If you did not, be prepared to justify this – you may have to admit that the failure to do so was an oversight and a learning point in its own right. This should help you think about your own experience and formulate your own answer. Here are a few examples of mistakes that could be used:'

- Incorrectly titrating intravenous midazolam during sedation and having to use a reversal drug.

- Discharging a patient with inappropriate medication. You may have spotted the mistake yourself and recalled the patient, or the mistake may have been spotted because the patient turned up a few days later with a more severe problem.

- Failing to plan for a potential complication prior to performing a procedure, as a result of which you were not prepared when it did happen. You then had to call for help to resolve the problem. For this mistake to be effective, you will need to discuss a complication that you should have planned for but somehow didn't. If no one ever plans for it because it is rare, then it isn't really a mistake.

- Failing to take into account a patient's comorbidities (perhaps you were in a hurry, or the notes were so thick that you made assumptions).

The above mistakes are all of a clinical nature. There are other mistakes you can discuss, which are of a managerial or communication nature. These include:

- Delegating a task to a colleague, assuming that they would know what to do and how to do it. They didn't and, as a result, patient care was delayed and/or confusion ensued, e.g. a junior dentist or student being left to take out a distoangular third molar and decoronating it, rendering salvage of the situation a little more difficult!

- Communicating important information to a patient, assuming they would understand it, when in fact they did not. As a result, they did not comply with your instructions. This could be because you were falsely reassured by their behaviour towards you or because you forgot to check their understanding, e.g. use of topical steroids in lichen planus, compliance with splint therapy in TMD.

- Being a bit too direct with a patient, not realising that in fact they were very sensitive. As a result, you risked causing them more distress than intended or compromising their trust in you.

At an interview, you can mention any mistake, unless the interviewers have directed you towards one particular type. For example, if simply asked for "a mistake", you could mention a clinical or non-clinical mistake. If asked specifically for a clinical mistake, then you would need to find a clinical scenario; fobbing off the interviewers by presenting a non-clinical scenario would result in a low mark. If in doubt, ask them.

Some interviewers will ask for a *recent* example. This usually means from within the last 6 to 12 months.

Playing safe vs. taking risks

Having viewed the feedback received by hundreds of candidates over dozens of specialties, we can comfortably say that those who score the highest on this question are candidates who present mistakes where they were actively involved and from which they will have learnt a lot from a personal point of view.

Before the interview, you must decide whether you wish to play safe, by presenting an average mistake or a non-clinical mistake, thereby guaranteeing yourself half the marks; or whether you want to be more daring, by presenting a more dramatic mistake, which, although risky, may yield you much higher marks if you can explain it properly using the steps highlighted earlier.

Remember to ensure that you demonstrate:

1. Personal learning and growth, e.g. how your practice has changed as a result
2. Institutional learning, e.g. did you discuss this at a clinical governance meeting, does it form a mainstay of your teaching to junior staff, or did it result in development of a protocol and guideline?

Employers and training programmes don't want people who never make mistakes. By definition, those people never do anything! What specialties are looking for is people who are open and honest about their mistakes, exercise duty of candour, and translate their learning into personal growth and lasting changes for the department, the institution and potentially the specialty as a whole. Think of all the developments in dentistry, e.g. side-vented needles in endodontics, cone-beam computed tomography (CBCT) in third molar assessment, etc. They are a direct result of learning from mistakes and complications and a desire to do better, and have left a lasting impact on the dental specialties they affected!

8.18 Describe a situation when you demonstrated professional integrity as a dentist

Many candidates have little understanding of the word "integrity", which then leads to poorly positioned answers. Integrity is a crucial part of the GDC's *Standards for the Dental Team*, and you should therefore show a good understanding, not only of the concept, but also of how it impacts on your work on a daily basis.

Integrity in your day-to-day work

Integrity refers to your ability to do the right thing when it may be tempting to react unethically for the sake of an easier life. This may be:

- Situations where you have made a mistake, where you would be expected to own up to it and take corrective action (see previous question)

- Situations where you should know how to handle a particular issue but somehow you don't. Integrity is about admitting your lack of knowledge and working towards addressing it (a lack of integrity would be pretending that you know what to do, which may put your patients and colleagues at risk)

- Situations where you discover that something is wrong and where you take proactive steps to address the situation (for example, if you discover that one of your colleagues has made a mistake, is an alcoholic, takes drugs, has abused a patient or is underperforming/incompetent)

- Situations where you were pressurised to do something that you knew or felt was wrong and where you resisted the pressure (e.g. a relative, a friend or a colleague encouraging you to breach patient confidentiality or a patient wanting you to carry out treatment that you know would not work or was not in their best interests, for financial gain)

- A colleague who wanted a favour that would place you in a difficult position (covering up for a mistake they made, etc)

The STAR approach provides a clear structure for the story. Each step is properly explained from the candidate's point of view, and there is a good level of reflection at the end. The example also clearly shows the candidate as someone who took responsibility for sorting the problem out, highlighting, where appropriate, how professional integrity was maintained.

Situation/Task "In my DCT job in oral surgery, a patient attended, referred for removal of a lower third molar. She gave a history of having occasional pain, which she described as 'twinges' but with no clear history of pericoronitis or episodes of antibiotics being prescribed. Her panoramic radiograph showed a possible intimate relationship of the roots of the tooth with the inferior alveolar nerve. She was insistent on having the third molar removed.

The patient was placing a lot of pressure to dictate treatment and demanding removal of the third molar. I spent quite a bit of time explaining to her that she didn't meet the NICE guidance for removal of the tooth and that there was no associated pathology, and that symptoms would likely settle. She indicated very strongly that she felt that I had not been trained properly and that any good dentist would just carry out the third molar removal. She demanded to see my consultant.

Action The patient was placing me under a lot of pressure to give her what she wanted, by attempting to intimidate me. It was important that I kept my cool and did not give in simply to get rid of the problem that I was facing. I provided her with valid reason, written advice on third molar surgery and NICE guidance and told her that I would arrange for my consultant to review her. I stressed that her third molar was high risk, given the appearances on the radiograph, and not without potential complications. My consultant concurred with my opinion, but offered a follow-up with the patient and the less invasive treatment option of an operculectomy. With a reiteration of the explanation, the patient left satisfied, feeling that she could return if her symptoms progressed.

Result/Reflect The patient went on to have no further symptoms and later on attended the department for an unrelated problem and took the time to thank me for saving her from a potentially unnecessary procedure. In this situation, I maintained my integrity in remaining professional in my relationship with the patient, despite the pressure that she was placing on me, by not giving into a request that I deemed to be against her best interests. It also helped dissipate her anxiety and maintain my credibility by involving a senior colleague appropriately. This example also illustrates the importance of communication in dealing with potential conflicts. In this case, by remaining civil, I avoided a potential complaint."

○ prescribing Abx · Following
SDCEP guidelines need dys Puc
dyn g infection.

↓

○ pulpitis episodes
· Xla s's + pt demanding abx.

8.19 What are the advantages and disadvantages of admitting when mistakes are made?

This question not only tests your integrity, but also your understanding of why integrity matters. The question looks very theoretical, calling for a list that you could simply learn and regurgitate; however, obviously, many candidates will come up with a similar list, and you therefore need to set yourself apart from the rest by bringing your personal experiences into your answer.

Advantages of admitting when mistakes are made

- You are able to repair the mistake much more quickly because you can involve others in the process.
- You can openly identify areas of possible improvement and gain support from your superiors to deal with them.
- You may originally annoy people, but they would be grateful for your honesty. In the long term, owning up to your mistakes may encourage people to trust you more because they know that you are honest.
- If you cover up a mistake for a long time and it is then discovered, the patient may lose trust in you and in the dental profession as a whole. You may be sued or struck off. If you admit the mistake and apologise early enough, the matter is much more likely to be resolved without such drastic consequences.

Disadvantages of admitting when mistakes are made

- Your colleagues and patients may form a lower opinion of you.
- You may be sacked, sued or struck off, or all of the aforementioned.
- Patients may lose trust towards you and/or the dental profession.

Generally speaking, the rule is that mistakes are forgivable, but dishonesty and misrepresentation almost never are. Not only are these fundamental probity issues for your governing body (the GDC) and the profession as a whole, behaviours such as these tarnish your reputation indefinitely and indelibly.

Bringing examples into your answer

As mentioned earlier, it is crucial that you mention examples in order to make your answer more personal and more interesting; otherwise, it will resemble everyone else's answer. When you give examples, keep your descriptions to two or three sentences. Here are a few effective examples:

"One of the advantages of admitting that you have made a mistake is that you can avoid complaints or at least minimise their impact. For example, in an orthodontic clinic post-orthognathic surgery, I once saw a patient who had some lower limb pain. I put it down to muscular cramp, but it took a chance encounter with the maxillofacial surgeon on the way out to diagnose a deep venous thrombosis. The parents were understandably upset, but I apologised and explained what had happened and the patient received treatment in a timely manner."

"Admitting to a mistake is helpful in maintaining a good relationship with patients, providing the communication with the patient is well handled. At the same time, it also helps in gaining support from your superiors to acquire new skills. I was asked to perform an incisional biopsy of a tongue lesion. Unfortunately, I was a little too superficial, and the reporting pathologist gave an equivocal report, as she was limited by the insufficient specimen my biopsy I had provided. This necessitated the biopsy being repeated. I immediately explained to the patient what had happened and apologised for any pain and inconvenience. She was very understanding and agreed to re-attend for the biopsy. I made my seniors aware of my error and arranged some further biopsies on a minor oral surgery list, for me to undertake them under supervision."

"A possible disadvantage of owning up to your mistakes is that the patient may lose trust in you as a dentist when they learn the truth. I remember a particular example of a situation where I had misplaced a blood sample for a patient and had to take a second one to replace it. Because it was something that was very simple and harmless, I hadn't felt it necessary to tell the patient about the mistake. The patient later came to know about it from a nurse who, as a gesture of goodwill, had asked the patient if she felt okay about the problem. Luckily, the patient was very understanding and let the matter go, but I could sense that I had bruised our relationship slightly as a result of my lack of attention to detail. I have worked hard to ensure this does not happen again."

To have an effective answer, all you need are three or four points with a couple of good examples. There is no need to give an example for every single point that you make; illustrating a couple of your points would be sufficient to provide a good balance. Don't be afraid of examples referring to negative consequences, but make sure they illustrate the point without presenting you as useless at your job (see the last example above).

8.20 How do you organise your workload?

At first glance, the question seems straightforward. However, like all questions relating to a generic topic, there is a risk that everyone ends up giving the same answer. You should therefore personalise it by giving suitable examples from your experience in order to stand out, even if the question does not explicitly ask for examples.

Organising your workload

Before you can answer the question effectively, you must identify the different ways in which you organise yourself at work. Don't try to be theoretical and second-guess a list of ways in which one might organise oneself. Simply think about what you do every day at work (it will make it easier to find suitable examples when you deliver the answer).

Here are a few examples that may be relevant to your situation, which you could describe:

- Making lists of patients and a list of tasks, whether patient-related or not. Prioritising your tasks

- Identifying whether you might require assistance from other people and ensuring they are briefed early enough (and available!)

- Reviewing your list on a regular basis, updating patient details and reprioritising if necessary

- Delegating tasks to the appropriate colleague / sharing the workload

- Working efficiently, by initiating investigations you need to do as early as possible in order to ensure that the results are back in time for when you need them

- Ensuring that you have the capacity to handle emergencies, first by building up some slack into your schedule if you can do that. Should something happen, you will then have time to catch up on the delay that occurs. Second, by identifying who is available for help if needed

- Making sure you plan your work in advance as much as you can, for example by reserving slots for specific matters (paperwork, teaching sessions, important meetings) as these may impose constraints onto your schedule; arranging for cross-cover when needed

Tools that you may use to support this

As well as discussing how you organise yourself, you could enrich your answer by mentioning the tools that you use to manage your work. These may include:

- PDA to keep track of patients
- Spreadsheet or word processor, e.g. for lists
- Electronic diary
- Secretary – this allows you to sell your team-playing abilities

Formulating an answer

A good answer will consist of three or four points, discussed in separate paragraphs/sections, each of which should contain a personal example in order to avoid simply listing the same items as everyone else. For example, instead of saying "I make a list of patients and prioritise them", "I delegate tasks to nurses and juniors", etc, you can present a more developed and personal answer by saying something along the following lines:

> "Before the clinic, I review all patients' notes, determining what I require for each encounter, e.g. study models and stainless steel crowns. At the start of the clinic, I have a discussion with my colleagues about how we can divide the patients according to skill mix, learning needs, etc. We also decide who will see any "walk-in" emergency patients during that session. I make sure that I request all laboratory work and write referral letters as I go along, to ensure that this is fresh in my mind. I update my job list throughout the day, to take account of developments. During my DFT placement in practice, I found it useful to allocate a specific slot every day to carry out all administrative tasks, usually before the clinical activity commenced, as I was least likely to be disturbed."

You can discuss the tools that you use, either as a separate section in your answer or by mixing the information with your examples. Whenever you mention a tool, explain not just that it is useful but also why it is useful. For example, "I regularly use a spreadsheet" is informative, but if many people say that, then there is little information to distinguish between all of you. You could rephrase this statement as follows:

> "I regularly use a spreadsheet on the practice computer for multi-stage treatment plans and any associated laboratory work for my patients. As well as helping me keep the information securely in one place, it enables me to have rapid access to all essential information. It also enables me to keep a rolling tab on laboratory fees and outstanding costs relating to the treatment plan."

8.21 How do you handle stress?

This is another generic question, where there is a risk of giving the same answer as hundreds of other candidates and, therefore, where you need to illustrate each point with personal examples in order to stand out. The marking schedule for this question will typically be rewarding:

- The variety of ways in which you can deal with stress
- Your ability to identify that you are getting stressed
- Your ability to show the relevance of the information to your work (i.e. by bringing personal examples, and, in the case of your hobbies, by explaining what you gain from them)

Many candidates fall into the trap of concentrating on their hobbies. In reality, interviewers will be looking for a broad range of ways of dealing with stress, including in the workplace. Note that the question does not explicitly ask how you recognise that you are stressed; however, it is a sad fact that many marking schemes allocate marks for relevant information that is not always explicitly requested. When in doubt, you should aim to provide an answer that is as complete as possible, by looking beyond the exact wording of the question and providing other relevant information. If your interviewers are helpful, they may prompt you for that information; others have higher expectations and may not be so kind.

Handling stress

There are different types of stress to which you may be exposed, both at work and in your personal life. Depending on the type of stress that you are facing, you will react and cope differently. This may include:

For stress caused by busy situations (e.g. being overworked):
- Taking a step back
- Remaining calm
- Organising your work, prioritising and delegating
- Trying to anticipate difficult periods and planning accordingly
- Taking appropriate breaks
- Breaking tasks off into smaller, more manageable chunks
- Asking for help from your colleagues
- Communicating well with others (e.g. maintaining momentum in a team, to ensure full coordination)
- Managing others' expectations (for example, if you are prioritising, inevitably someone's main priority will become bottom of your list. Not managing their expectations would potentially result in a conflict)

For stress of a more emotional nature (e.g. difficulty in dealing with negative issues such as personality clashes, unexpected adverse outcomes or complications from treatment plans, high expectations from others, feeling of powerlessness)
- Sharing your problems with colleagues
- Discussing problems with your friends and family

For general stress (e.g. accumulation of fatigue)
- Socialising with colleagues or friends
- Having time for yourself, hobbies, centres of interest outside of dentistry

Rather than simply list some of the above items, you should focus your answer on your personal experience, explaining how you deal with a range of different situations that you commonly face in the workplace. Since the question is not specifically relating to the workplace, you may also mix in some information relating to other settings, if you feel that they are appropriate.

Example of an effective answer

"I deal with stress differently, depending on the situation. For example, during my orthodontic DCT clinics, I often have to deal with multiple unplanned emergency attendances on my own, some of which can take a long time to handle. In such circumstances, I find it very useful to take stock of the situation once the most urgent matters have been attended to. This ensures that I remain in control of the situation and do not miss any important tasks. If I feel that an issue may cause problems later on, I keep in touch with my trainer so that he is aware of the situation and able to provide input, as needed. I also work closely with the dental nurses and orthodontic therapists, because they are invaluable in getting some of the tasks done very efficiently and often provide very useful information that I can use to make more informed decisions for our patients. When I am very busy, I try to take a short break to have a coffee. I find that having regular breaks really helps to keep me focused.

"When I worked in paediatric dentistry, I found many families had unreasonably high expectations; this could be stressful at times. Although I could see that they had their child's best interest at heart, I found they were often keen to blame the dental profession for their child's poor oral hygiene or caries, which could more easily be linked to poor dietary choices at home. This created a sometimes very negative and stressful atmosphere. Generally speaking, I was able to deal with this, because I felt that they reacted in this way as a result of a natural concern for their child. It can be very useful to discuss problems with colleagues as it provides an opportunity to share the problem with someone else but also to understand how *they* deal with similar issues. Often, we both learn from these conversations and I have found that, since I have been talking to them in this

---

way, they have started to do the same with me. This has led to better team working, which has further reduced stress.

"I think that the key to a stress-free life is to make sure that you are properly conditioned to deal with problems. I have often found that I react much more calmly to problems when I have had the opportunity to relax outside of work. Personally, I enjoy playing sport with friends, particularly cricket. I also enjoy reading books such as crime novels and history books. I find that, by combining group and personal activities, I strike a good balance in my leisure time, which then makes it easier to deal with stress generally.

"Friends and colleagues often comment that I am a relaxed individual, but I know that stress is beginning to affect me if I start to find it difficult to think straight, or if I become irritable or disorganised. When I recognise this, I make sure that I set aside some valuable relaxation time, usually in the evening, to stop letting the stress get to me."

8.22 How do you recognise that you are stressed?

Ways in which you can recognise that you are stressed include:

Behavioural effects

- Feeling tired, tense, irritable or anxious
- Poor concentration; becoming forgetful; making small/silly mistakes
- Difficulty in dealing calmly with everyday pressures
- Loss of appetite / too much appetite
- Working shorter or longer hours
- Poor time management or punctuality
- Shorter fuse; increased tension and conflict with colleagues or patients

Physical effects

- Lower resistance to infection
- Raised heart rate
- Aching neck and shoulder
- Headaches
- Insomnia

Note: this is not a clinical question on the manifestations of stress, so there is no need to become highly detailed by mentioning some recognised but less appealing symptoms such as "blurred vision" or "dizziness", which could impair your ability to be safe at work.

Avoid listing a number of points, as this will make your answer bland. Draw upon real situations where you became stressed in the past, explain how you identified that you were stressed and then briefly explain how you dealt with that stress. The emphasis should be on stress recognition rather than stress resolution here, though you should ensure that you mention both, as both are likely to appear in the marking scheme.

8.23 Give an example of a stressful situation in which you have been involved

This question is testing your ability to deal with pressure and stress by means of an example. Through discussing the example, you will be expected to explain which demands were made on you personally and how you coped/dealt with them.

Which examples can you discuss?

Try to choose a complex enough scenario where you were really stressed, otherwise you will struggle to explain the issue convincingly and to demonstrate your full skill set. This may include situations where you had to:

- Deal with several tasks at the same time, e.g. several emergencies, urgent requests or tasks with tight deadlines
- Do something that was unfamiliar and which you were under pressure to deliver quickly
- Deal with a difficult or abusive patient who was taking your time, putting you behind in the rest of your work
- Work with a colleague who was difficult or unhelpful
- Deal with the workload of one or several absent colleagues with little or no senior availability
- Negotiate with a colleague who disagreed with your approach, when you had little time to argue

Delivering the answer

Once you have settled on one example, identify the skills and behaviours that you exhibited to deal with the situation and avoid/deal with your stress. For example, if you had to deal with a multitasking situation, then you will inevitably have to mention:

- How you prioritised the patients and shared the workload with colleagues to resolve the situation
- How you ensured that you maintained good communication
- How you gained support from seniors
- How, maybe, you negotiated with colleagues to make room for small breaks for yourself and others

If you had to deal with a difficult patient, you will talk about how you ensured you remained calm, used all your communication skills to establish a rapport and deal with the patient, and maybe involved other team members to help you out.

Don't lose sight of the fact that the question is about the stress incurred during the scenario and not just about the situation itself. This means that you must go into detail about what demands, pressure and stress you faced, what *you* did, and how it helped resolve the problem and reduce your stress level.

Concluding the answer

Conclude your answer by explaining what happened at the end and, if appropriate, how you relaxed when you went back home (had a bath, relaxed with family, played table tennis with friends, etc) to provide a complete answer.

If the situation provided an opportunity to learn from it and develop new skills and behaviours, then you should mention that. For example, after dealing with a difficult patient, you might have debriefed with a senior colleague and discussed alternative approaches. You might even have agreed to develop your skills further by going on a communication skills course. Similarly, after dealing with multiple emergencies or a difficult on-call, you might have sought advice from senior colleagues and learnt about other ways of working. Basically, if there is an opportunity to learn, make sure you mention and present yourself as someone who is always trying to improve and develop.

If the stress was due to a systemic problem (e.g. an inefficient system, the absence of the right equipment, the short-notice unavailability of staff) then you could also explain how you tried to change the system once the event was over (e.g. introducing a new proforma, arranging a team meeting to discuss the problem), as a means to prevent the stressful situation from recurring.

8.24 Describe a situation when you have used a holistic approach in managing a patient

What the interviewers are looking for

The question asks you to discuss how you have used a holistic approach as part of a real-life scenario. In your answer, you will be expected to describe, through the use of a specific personal example, how you identified and addressed the physical, social and psychological needs of a patient.

This may seem like stating the obvious, but it frames the question, and without considering the answer in this way, you will not score well. The key to this question is really to find a good example that enables you to demonstrate your experience and ability in applying all three aspects in the management of a single patient.

Note that the question asks for a clinical situation. It does not mean you have to go into vast clinical detail but simply that it must be related to a patient at work, rather than, say, a friend with whom you might have dealt.

Examples you can discuss

Your example must describe your care of a patient and must include all of the aforementioned areas. This could include:

- A patient to whom you broke bad news
- A patient whose lifestyle was impacting on their oral health
- A patient who was finding it difficult to cope with their diagnosis
- A patient with psychological factors or functional overlay, key to their diagnosis and management, e.g. atypical facial pain, burning mouth syndrome
- A patient with multiple comorbidities impacting upon treatment modality

Use the STAR structure (see 5.2)

Situation/Task	Describe the type of patient and how they presented to you.
Action	Explain how you recognised and addressed the patient's different needs.
Result/Reflect	Explain how the patient was helped with your approach (grateful, much-improved lifestyle, got a new job and sorted

> themselves out, etc). Explain what you feel you did well and, if prompted, what you could have done better.

Try to be as practical as you can, describing what you actually did to address the patient's needs. Too many candidates offer statements such as: "I identified the patient's psychological needs and addressed them appropriately".

This only explains what needs you identified, but it would be interesting to know what those needs exactly were and how they were addressed. For example, the patient may have had a need for psychological support; consequently, you discussed support groups and gave the patient leaflets to read and websites to visit.

The different needs

Physical needs
Describe the physical needs of the patient and how you addressed them. In this section try to give just enough detail to clearly communicate that you were competent burning mouth syndrome but do not overdo it on the clinical detail – this is not the purpose of the question. In some cases, your answers could even be as simple as referring the patient to a specialist or to a senior colleague. All that matters is that you have addressed the needs in a sensible manner.

Social needs
Describe the social needs of the patient. Were there any issues precluding regular attendance for dental review/treatment? Were there any issues in terms of financial constraints that required a modification of the treatment plan? Were there lifestyle modifications that the patient required help with, e.g. smoking/alcohol cessation advice and help? Did you enlist the help of some members of the multidisciplinary team to sort out some of the issues (e.g. general medical practitioner)? Did you provide leaflets / written information to the patient?

Psychological needs
Describe the psychological needs of the patient. Did they need support in coming to terms with a difficult diagnosis? Did they need counselling? Did they need mental health input coordinated by their general medical practitioner? Was there a considerable amount of "functional overlay" impairing their ability and/or altering their perception of their diagnosis (e.g. "catastrophising")?

8.25 Describe a time when you had to deal with a sceptical patient

This is another question asking for an example, and which you will therefore need to answer using the STAR approach (see 5.2). This question is primarily about communication, the respect of others and, in some cases, teamwork (e.g. if you needed to involve input from other people to help you resolve the situation).

What the interviewers are looking for

The main criteria that the interviewers will be looking for include:

Communication
- Listening to the patient's point of view, exploring the patient's concerns and addressing any underlying issues; for example, if they distrust an orthodox treatment plan, you should investigate why.

- Communication with the patient in a way they can understand (basic English if needed, interpreter, diagrams) and that they have time to digest the information and ask questions to you or others.

- Ensuring that the patient receives all the information that you can give them. This could be through the involvement of other professionals (for example, by involving another colleague, a nurse or referring to a suitable specialist) or by giving a patient information leaflet (PIL).

Teamwork
Asking a senior colleague or other member of the team for advice on how you should handle the situation, or asking them to intervene, if necessary.

Respect for patient's autonomy
The patient has the right to make a decision for themselves. If, in your example, your patient still disagreed with you despite your best efforts, don't panic – this may be a powerful example; what matters is how you dealt with it. It is a patient's right to disagree and your duty to accept that they can do so. In such cases, it is important to have demonstrated that they understood what the consequences might be for them and what other options were available. It is also important to mention that you documented the essence of the conversation and the decision.

Examples you can discuss

There are many reasons for a patient to be sceptical. Here are a few examples that you may have encountered recently:

- They do not trust you for one reason or another. Maybe they have prior bad experiences with friends or relatives, which would make them doubt your word.

- They may have gained information from the media (for example, through TV, newspapers or the Internet) that gives them a different perspective.

- They may be more informed than the average patient (e.g. scientists, clinicians), requiring tailored information and having an altered perspective.

- They may have personal beliefs (against conventional treatment, for example) or simply a language problem.

- Your explanations or proposed management options may be different from their expectations.

Once you have found the right example, describing the situation is fairly straightforward using the STAR technique (see 5.2).

8.26 Outline a time when you had to support a colleague with a work-related problem

Although the topic raised by the question is that of a colleague in difficulty, this is not a question about how to deal with a difficult colleague or an unsafe colleague. It is really a question about support, and therefore communication and teamwork, so you should ensure that your answer focuses on these two skills.

The type of situations where you may have needed to support a colleague with a work-related problem may include:

A busy colleague who finds it hard to find time to study

You would discuss the situation with the colleague and perhaps offer to take on some of their tasks, when appropriate, to relieve them from the pressure they face. If they are busy because they are not very efficient, you may offer to help them out by showing them how they can plan and organise their work better (making sure you are not patronising them in doing so). If you are also studying for exams, you may consider supporting them by pairing up with them to revise together. If you have already passed the exam they are studying for, you could organise informal teaching/support sessions to help them out.

A colleague who lacks knowledge or experience and struggles

First, you must make sure your colleague is not performing tasks beyond their level of competence. You can encapsulate this in your answer by stating that your priority would be to ensure the highest standard of patient care and safety. Many people have small knowledge-based sticking points, which they feel stupid asking about because they feel they should know them. If this is the case, you could give a brief explanation or tutorial and then explain how you learned this and if there are good books or web resources that you use when you are stuck. This encourages them to try to look things up themselves the next time they are stuck.

If the issue is the need to learn a practical skill, see if it is something you can go over in a skills lab together – you may find that there is a simple step that is being forgotten, and this is a very easy environment to iron this out. If it is more complex, you could recommend the course that you did to learn the skill, or set up some ward-based mentorship for the skill. If you know that the task in question is being performed, then you could encourage your colleague to be there when it happens and ideally adjust the rota so that they have an opportunity to reinforce their learning of that skill with practical experience.

The basis of your answer is that you would support your colleague, making sure that they are not exposed to situations where they feel stupid or dangerous, and encourage them to improve their knowledge or skills to overcome any deficiency.

A colleague in a personality clash with another colleague

Dealing with personality clashes from an external perspective is always dangerous because you risk making matters worse by appearing to take sides. Supporting your colleague may consist of listening to them and allowing them to vent their frustration, so they know that they can share their problem with someone else. This may help your colleague put things in perspective and discuss the issue with their colleague directly. If the clash is with someone more senior, then you may encourage your colleague to discuss the problem with another senior colleague whom they trust (e.g. a consultant, their educational supervisor). Essentially, you would ensure that you are there for them without necessarily getting directly involved yourself in resolving the matter. You are *supporting* your colleague, not *replacing* them.

A colleague who finds it hard to remain motivated in their job

You must never lose sight of the fact that you are supporting your colleague and not seeking to dictate a course of action to them. Supporting them may involve sitting down with them to help them understand why they are not motivated. Perhaps they are not getting enough support from senior colleagues, in which case you may want to encourage them to raise the issue with their educational supervisor. Perhaps they are doing an attachment in a specialty that does not interest them, in which case you may wish to discuss with them how they can make the attachment more interesting or help them understand the importance or advantages of their current job in their long-term career plan; perhaps you would encourage them to get involved in a project such as an audit, to give them a sense of purpose.

A colleague who is being bullied by a senior colleague

Bullying is not acceptable in any environment but, whilst you may want to try to resolve the issue yourself, you should try to take the part of a supportive friend and aim to maintain an objective view. Direct involvement on your part should be a last resort.

Your support should begin by simply listening to your colleague and helping them think about the problem rather than getting involved yourself – it will help you to establish their side of the story. If you felt that patient care was being compromised and that your colleague was unable to deal with the problem, then you would need to raise the matter with a senior colleague. If you can, avoid discussing topics involving drink, drugs or bullying, unless the interviewers specifically ask you about them (we will see how to handle difficult colleagues later on), as this takes the attention away from the support towards your colleague and it may lead to answers that are potentially controversial.

Note that the question is asking for a work-related problem and not a personal problem. However, in some circumstances, the two will be inextricably linked (i.e. problems such as a sick child, marital problems or even train delays may have an impact on work-related performance). You can therefore mention in your answer how you sought to support your colleague in relation to more personal problems, but only to the extent that they are impacting on their work, and providing they do not form the main thread of your answer; otherwise, your answer will be off-topic and your score will be accordingly low.

Delivering the answer

Since the question is asking for a specific example, you should make sure that you do not speak generically about how you would support a colleague but that you provide an example of a specific situation.

You should structure your answer using the STAR approach (see 5.2), explaining first the nature of the problem from your colleague's point of view (i.e. setting out why he/she was in need of support), explaining how you supported him, and how the story ended (hopefully your actions led to a positive outcome).

Be prepared to answer a follow-up question on what you could have done better. There is no need to volunteer this information unless they request it explicitly when probing.

8.27 What skills or personal attributes do you possess that will make you a good trainee in this specialty?

This is a very broad question, which leaves many candidates perplexed simply because they don't know where to start.

Where are the marks?

For this type of question, the marking scheme will reward:

- Your understanding of the specialty and the training
- Your ability to list skills and attributes relevant to the specialty
- Your ability to demonstrate, with full use of your personal experience, that you possess those skills and attributes
- The clarity of your answer (which will come from the structure of your answer and the concise nature of your examples)

Which skills and attributes can you mention?

The answer very much depends on the person specification for your specialty and grade. When you face such a question, you can talk about pretty much what you want, providing you respect the following rules:

- Ensure that the skills and attributes mentioned cover a wide enough spectrum. You should consult the person specification to understand the requirements that your interviewers will be testing.

- Choose a maximum of four skills and attributes. Although the person specification may cover a lot more than four, you cannot possibly talk about all of them in two minutes; otherwise, you will remain very superficial. Give priority to those for which you can more easily demonstrate your suitability, experience and strengths.

- Choose skills and attributes that are strongly linked to the specialty, and order them in decreasing order of importance. For example, being empathetic and a good listener are both important in most specialties but, in some specialties, other skills are more prominently used.

- Structure your answer on a skill-by-skill basis. Mention one skill/attribute, and explain why it is important for the specialty. Give examples from your experience to back up your claims.

- Make sure that you are specific in the description of the skills and attributes that you choose to present. For example, "I am a good communicator" is vague. A punchier statement would be "I am a good communicator and, in particular, I am very effective at dealing with conflict between other team members or in situations where I need to negotiate with others." The more specific you are, the more impact you will have, and the easier it will be to find suitable examples to illustrate your purpose.

- If you can, try to group several skills in one point, if they are related. For example, you may want to say that you are good at making decisions and that you call for help when necessary and that you are a good team player. These could constitute three different points, but you could also raise all of them in one single point, with a sentence such as: "I am very good at making decisions when faced with difficult situations and I am always prepared to ask for help, if required. I am also very good at implementing my decisions by communicating with the relevant colleagues and delegating responsibilities appropriately" (you can then follow this with an example). This approach gives more body to your answer.

Examples of structures for different specialties

Oral surgery

Example 1
- Good manual dexterity and hand–eye coordination
- Good ability to keep calm under pressure and make sensible decisions (including seeking help from others if necessary)
- Very good at engaging with patients, explaining procedures and providing reassurance when necessary
- Good team-working abilities, in particular: good relationships with all team members and wider multidisciplinary team; good ability to interface with other specialties

Example 2
- Patient, able to remain calm under pressure and to take initiative in challenging situations
- Able to make decisions and resolve complex issues, calling for help if required
- Good at engaging with people at all levels, whether they are patients, junior colleagues or senior colleagues
- Committed to hard work, enjoy volunteering for new projects and willing to learn from own experience

Orthodontics

Example 1

- Good communication skills, able to address a wide range of people with different levels of understanding and different cultural backgrounds
- Confident in addressing complex issues and able to think laterally to find solutions to problems
- Capacity to work well in a multidisciplinary team and see the viewpoints of others, to benefit patient care and outcomes
- Able to manage time and prioritise tasks and commitments

Example 2

- Relates easily to a wide range of people, whether they are patients or other members of the dental team, both in the clinical and non-clinical environment
- Caring and supportive. Able to show empathy towards patients but also towards colleagues, volunteering to help when required
- Good analytical skills and good ability to make decisions, both independently and with senior advice, if required
- Organised and able to deal with difficult situations through teamwork, self-discipline and tenacity

Oral medicine

- Very good at considering a wide range of possibilities and thinking laterally, to work through things from multiple different viewpoints
- Works well with allied health professionals, including the medical team, to ensure optimum patient care
- Inquisitive and sees questions and problems as challenges, both from an individual patient care perspective and a broader, research-oriented aspect
- Able to view patients holistically, with a strong sense of patients as people
- Very organised and thorough; able to work well under pressure, remain calm and take appropriate decisions, calling for help if necessary
- Good team player and, in particular, able to communicate well with colleagues at all levels; not afraid to discuss problems if necessary, even with seniors
- Empathic, good listener and able to engage quickly with patients

Special care dentistry

- Flexibility, decisiveness and resilience
- Remains calm under pressure and objective in emotive and/or pressurised situations

- Works well in a multidisciplinary team and interfaces meaningfully with other specialties
- Good ability to empathise and communicate under challenging circumstances with adults and adolescents with physical and/or mental disabilities
- Holistic approach to patients with complex needs

Paediatric dentistry

- Good listener, able to engage with patients, to reassure and empathise
- Quick thinking and able to deal well with pressure; good at making safe decisions quickly, asking for help from senior colleagues if required.
- Good at collaborating with a wide range of people; sensitive to the needs of the various members of the team

Delivering your answer

You can see from the above that many of the same skills and attributes are common in different answers. Indeed, in the person specifications for different dental specialties given in the recruitment round in 2019, the qualities sought were virtually identical. After all, there is only limited choice. You will not be judged on how different your answer sounds (i.e. you don't have to find some obscure skill to stand out), but on the completeness of your answer and the way in which you illustrate the points that you are making.

Once you have made a point (which may consist of several statements, as shown in each bullet point above), provide examples from your practice. It is best to avoid going into too much detail for the examples, as you only have 20 to 30 seconds per point. This can be achieved either by sticking to one example per point, which you briefly describe without going into too much detail (otherwise you won't have much time for other points; or by listing several general situations where you may have demonstrated the skill in question, explaining briefly afterwards how you handled the situation.

Example of an effective answer (partial – using one example only)

"I am patient, able to remain calm under pressure and to take the initiative in challenging situations. For example, recently I was confronted with an apprehensive patient in the walk-in dental service. I could see that he was becoming more agitated, and this in turn made him irritable, due to the long wait to be seen that evening. This caused him to become confrontational with the reception staff. I talked to the patient to try and persuade him to calm down. It took a while, but I was able to get to the bottom of the anxiety driving his

> behaviour, whilst at the same time remaining firm regarding the acceptability of his behaviour towards the staff."

You can see that the example is only briefly expanded upon, almost as a teaser for the interviewers. Their next question will then likely ask you to expand on the situation. Also, as this is only one point out of four, there is no time to dwell on the detail too much. The communication and teamwork aspects are emphasised just enough to make the point.

Example of an effective answer (partial – listing several examples)

"I feel that I am good at being versatile and considering many different viewpoints. Over the past few years, I have had the opportunity to exhibit problem solving under controlled conditions, in consultant-led oral medicine clinics, where the diagnoses are often far from straightforward. In addition, I often contribute meaningfully to treatment planning for orthodontic patients in my current role as a DCT within the department. There are often many different angles and perspectives and no clear right answer, with factors such as patient compliance, expectations, wishes and understanding all coming into play. I feel that I understand patients holistically and am able to juggle all these balls in the air, whilst making good treatment decisions."

Again, there is no time to go into any detail. What you are trying to achieve is a demonstration, to your panel, of where and how you use the skill stated, with a view that, if they are interested, they may ask for more detail about any particular example.

8.28   **What are your main strengths?**

This question is in fact the same one as 8.27. Your main strengths should be the skills and attributes that make you suitable for the specialty, and there is therefore no reason why you should be providing a different answer. Other questions that can be answered in a similar fashion include:

- How would your colleagues describe you?
- What would your friends say about you?
- What would you like your consultant to write in your reference?
- If I looked at your multi-source feedback, what would it say? (Stay away from any negative feedback unless they ask)
- What makes you a good dentist?
- What would you like written in your obituary?

What if they only ask for a single strength?

It may be that the question is worded in the singular, i.e. "What would you consider to be your single biggest strength?" If this happens, then the approach to the question is the same, except that you will need to place your entire focus on just one of the four points that you would normally mention.

There is one trick, though, that will enable you to sell a bit more than just one point: it is to simply list a range of points in the first sentence before zooming in on the main point that you want to talk about. It would give something like:

> "Well, I have many strengths, including being organised, able to work well under pressure, being a good team player and a good colleague. However, if I had to choose a single strength, I would say that it is my ability to communicate well with people at all levels, even in conflicting situations."<then illustrate with examples>

8.29 What is your main weakness?

This question is often a worry for candidates, who fear that they may sound too clichéd or uninteresting by using a weakness that the interviewers are likely to have heard several times that day.

What is this question about?

Contrary to some of the interview myths that circulate, this question is NOT about demonstrating that you are perfect and that you have no weaknesses. On the contrary, the interviewers will be testing your honesty, your insight, your ability to learn from your mistakes/problems and to develop as an individual. Rather like the question on a mistake that you made (see 8.17), they expect you to talk openly about your own failures – an honest clinician is a safe one, whom patients and colleagues can trust. So, don't be afraid to be personal, as this is the only way in which you can maximise your mark.

The weakness(es) should not be strengths in disguise but rather areas that you are aware of and account for. We have all worked with people who appear to have no insight into their weaknesses and the potential to be dangerous is considerable. If you have self-doubt, this can paralyse you with fear if it remains unchecked, but can be a valuable counterbalance to being over-confident if heeded to just the right degree.

Where do people go wrong when answering this question?

The problem does not lie so much in the weakness that candidates choose to mention in their answer, but in the way it is delivered. Most answers sound clichéd because candidates present the weakness in a simplistic, almost black-and-white manner. A common answer is of the format: "I can't say 'no', but I am aware of it and I am working on it." In such an answer, there is no attempt to explain exactly how they are dealing with it. This makes the answer very standard and totally uninteresting.

There is also no real attempt to explain in any detail what the impact of the weakness on the candidate is, for instance by providing an example which would lift any ambiguity. The lack of example means that the interviewers are left to extrapolate from the basic statement made by the candidate in any way they like, and the candidate therefore loses control over the way in which their message is received.

For example:
- "I can't say 'no'" may give the impression that you are weak.
- "I have high expectations of others" may give the impression that you are a control freak and unfriendly.

How to choose a good weakness

There are three parameters that you need to consider to choose a suitable weakness:

- Make sure that it is one of your real weaknesses, as you will be much more at ease talking about it in detail than if you make it up (answers that are faked tend to sound rehearsed, vague and clichéd).

- Choose a weakness that, in different circumstances, can be considered a strength. The strategy is to present the weakness as a strength that can sometimes become a problem.

- Choose a weakness that can be remedied. There are weaknesses that can be difficult to correct, such as being disorganised, or getting frustrated at certain events. These are best avoided.

Examples of weaknesses

There are numerous examples of weakness that you can use, some being more original and creative than others. It is important that you choose one that you are comfortable talking about, as most of the impact that you will have in delivering the answer rests in your tone of voice and general confidence.

If you are unsure as to which weakness to choose, try different examples and see which one sounds best. We have set out below a range of weaknesses, which you may want to consider, listing their negative and positive interpretations, together with some means of dealing with them. See if they are true to your situation and, if they are, adapt them to match your situation, bringing your own examples into the answer.

Being a perfectionist
This answer is probably one of most quoted at interviews, and one that is least likely to make you sound credible. By itself, it is not a bad weakness to mention but the interviewers will have heard it so many times in one day that you may just be subconsciously penalised for your lack of originality. If you want to use the "perfectionist" answer, we would advise you to find a more specific slant to the weakness so that you do not present it under such a broad heading. Some of the weaknesses have a "perfectionist" slant to them but sound less clichéd.

Finding it difficult to say "no"

This is also a commonly given answer, but perhaps a little less clichéd than the "perfectionist" answer, primarily because it has more words to it and therefore the impact is softened. If you want to use this weakness, you will need to convey the meaning of not being able to say "no", without actually using that phrase. For example: "There are times where I take on so many simultaneous projects that it can be difficult to juggle them all." The meaning is the same, but the wording is a bit more original.

Positive: You are a good team player, a good colleague, and always willing to help.

Negative: You may take on too much work and get stressed, or fail to deliver on some projects (hopefully minor ones!).

What you can do about it:

- Learn to become more assertive (more experience, or course).
- Learn to manage colleagues' expectations (so that they are okay about you saying "no").
- Work with colleagues to help them find alternative solutions.
- Be more realistic about your ability to deliver and more open with colleagues about issues.
- Be more proactive in delegating to others so that you can say "yes" without having to take on everything yourself.

Having high standards and a tendency to expect others to follow the same standards as you

Positive: Being driven, you have achieved a lot and you deliver results to your team above their expectations. You have also encouraged others in your team to achieve and they did well as a result. You are seen as a good motivator and a "doer".

Negative: Some of your colleagues may not be able to follow your pace. You are trying to impose methods and principles, which they may not adhere to, and this may cause friction at times (i.e. you risk being seen as controlling).

What you can do about it:

- Learn to be a bit more flexible with colleagues. Take the time to know them. It may give you ideas about how you can approach them.
- Ensure that all team members have been trained in the skills you are expecting them to perform.
- Be more open-minded in your approach and accept that others may have ideas which are as good as, if not better than, yours.

Having a direct style of communication

This weakness is probably not suitable for specialties where communication is an ultra-essential skill (such as paediatric dentistry or special care dentistry). However, if addressed properly, it can be used successfully for a wide range of dental specialties, from oral surgery to dental public health.

Positive: People know where they stand with you; they know that, if they ask for your opinion, they will get an answer that they can use towards their own thinking process. Generally, you find it easy to be trusted because people know that, if there is an issue, you will discuss it openly.

Negative: There are times when more subtlety and diplomacy are required, and you may encounter situations where communicating too openly may cause friction.

What you can do about it:
- Learn to appreciate the impact of your communication on others.
- Learn to recognise when you can be yourself and when you need to soften your style.
- Seek guidance from seniors; perhaps go on a course.

Finding it difficult to delegate

This weakness is the result of lack of experience of working in a delegation environment. This lack of experience, coupled with the fear that you may lose control of the situation, leads to your taking over the situation.

Positive: You deliver consistently good results and, in an environment where most people rotate frequently, it can be an asset not to overload new team members until they have established their ability.

Negative: People may see you as someone distant (sometimes). Also, by trying to do everything yourself, you end up having too much on your plate, with a risk of getting stressed.

What you can do about it:
- Be more attentive to juniors and find opportunities to delegate
- Get to know your colleagues early on, so that you find it easier to trust them and therefore delegate
- Discuss with your seniors and/or go on a course.

Having a tendency to take criticism or negative outcomes personally

This weakness can work well if you have the right type of personality.

Positive: Taking things personally pushes you to act on problems quickly.

Negative: Being over-negative may make you appear under-confident (and miserable).

What you can do about it:
- Discuss with colleagues and see how they deal with criticism, complaints and negative outcomes.
- Use every incident as an opportunity to learn.

Getting too involved with patients
This would refer to situations where patients have many issues, and where you find it difficult to put a stop to a consultation for fear of missing something out or upsetting the patient.

Positive: You are thorough and caring.

Negative: You can overrun and/or get stressed.

What you can do about it:
- Learn to become gently assertive.
- Discuss with colleagues to understand how they do address this issue.

Getting too attached to patients
This refers to situations where you are struggling to maintain the professional barrier in your dealings with a patient and push the empathy to a point where it personally affects you psychologically.

Positive: You are caring and empathetic.

Negative: You get stressed.

What you can do about it:
- Learn through experience to keep the appropriate distance.
- Discuss with colleagues/seniors.

Taking your worries home with you
This refers to situations where you finish your work and feel the need to double-check things when you get home or keep worrying about whether your instructions will be followed once you have left. In some cases, this may result in you having to call the clinic/department on days off, or even to stay late to ensure that things are done properly.

Positive: You are thorough and conscientious.

Negative: You may get stressed or even irritate others, who feel you don't trust them. It may also interfere with your social/private life.

What you can do about it:

- Optimise your communication with colleagues so that you can be sure they know what needs to be done.
- Discuss with colleagues how they deal with it.
- Set yourself lists of tasks and tick off when completed.
- Nominate an individual to email securely through nhs.net email address if there are outstanding jobs or queries you have when away from the workplace.

All these are examples, which will work well if they are explained in a personal manner. There are other approaches that you can adopt, but which, in our experience, are less successful. These include:

- Using a weakness that is not linked to personality but to something practical, such as lack of research. Most marking schemes would be based around a personality-based weakness, and therefore, using a more practical weakness may score lower. If you have any doubt, or if you are really keen to talk about a non-personality-related weakness, then there is no harm in asking the interviewers whether they want a personality-based weakness or whether you can use something relating to your training.

- Using a weakness that is in the past and already resolved. This does not answer the question, which is "What is your main weakness?". Using an old weakness would not demonstrate that you have any insight into your current behaviours and therefore may score lower. In answering this question, playing safe rarely pays off. There can be a benefit in taking risks.

Structure to answer the question

There are many ways in which you can answer this question; however, having heard thousands of people answering this question, both in our experience of interviewing and in our coaching experience, we have found the following structure to be one of the most effective:

Step 1:	**Quick positive introduction**, to place a positive context on the weakness (this must be no more than 15 seconds or so, otherwise you will give the impression that you are avoiding the question).

Step 2:	**State the weakness and explain the negative impact it has.** In doing so, ensure that you use words that do not make the weakness sound awful. "I can't delegate effectively" sounds bad, but "I sometimes find it difficult to delegate, particularly when working with new and less experienced colleagues" is more specific and more realistic too.
Step 3:	**Give a specific example** of a situation that illustrates the weakness. Spend some time on this section. The purpose of the example is to remove any doubt in the interviewers' minds about the seriousness of the weakness.
Step 4:	**Explain what you learnt from that situation.** This will enable the interviewers to visualise exactly how reflective you can be. This, together with the next step, is one of the most important parts of the answer.
Step 5:	**Explain how you attempt to deal with the weakness generally.** This will ensure that the interviewers tick the marking box that says "Takes concrete steps to remedy the weakness".

Example of an effective answer

It would take hundreds of pages to illustrate how each weakness can be discussed; however, once you have read the following sample answer, you will get the idea of how the above structure can be applied, and you will have no problem adapting it to your own experience and circumstances. I have chosen the weakness of "taking on too much" to demonstrate how you can build the answer using the different steps stated above.

Step 1	"I have always been an ambitious person and, as a result, I always show a lot of enthusiasm in getting involved in all sorts of projects. If you look at my CV, you will see that I have achieved a lot, not only in terms of clinical experience, but also in terms of audit and teaching experience.
Step 2	"However, there are times where I have been a little too greedy and became involved in too many projects at once, as a result of which I either placed myself under too much pressure, or I had to arrange an extension of the deadline.

Step 3   "One example that springs to mind is a situation that arose last year, when, as well as working in a busy Restorative DCT1 job in the dental hospital and studying hard for MJDF exams, I had agreed to deliver quarterly lectures to dental students, volunteered to do some number-crunching for my consultant's research project and also agreed to do two audits, one of which I was keen to lead throughout. After two months, I could see that I would never be able to complete all this before I moved to my next post, and so I had to go back to my consultant to explain that I could only do one of the audits.

Step 4   "I felt I had let down my colleagues in this particular instance, but it made me realise how crucial it is to be aware of your own capacities and that, although you may look good when you accept a project, it can cause problems if you don't deliver. On reflection, I also feel that I could have delivered as expected if I had thought about involving someone else when there was still time to do so, such as a dental student, who could have made a start on collecting the data.

Step 5   "I have become very aware of the problems associated with getting involved in too many projects and the impact both on myself and on other people. As a result, I try my best to think carefully before launching into new projects (without curbing my own enthusiasm, of course). I also try to involve others more when appropriate, which has the advantage of getting juniors involved in new projects too."

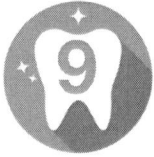

9 Academic and clinical governance questions

Questions on academic activities (e.g. teaching, research), or on clinical governance, are a component part of DCT and ST interviews. These can be generic (e.g. "What is clinical governance?") or specific (e.g. "How does risk management affect your daily practice?").

They are generally easier to prepare for than the more personal questions addressed in previous chapters, because they are factual and therefore rely, to a large extent, on information that you will have learnt before the interview. However, to achieve a high mark, repeating information learnt by heart will not be enough; you will be expected to reflect on your own experience and provide a more personal slant to the issues raised. This chapter will provide you with essential information, which you may need at your interview.

In some academic and clinical governance stations, you may be asked to discuss a paper that you have read recently; we would therefore advise you to read the journals appropriate for your preferred specialty before the interview, so that you can approach such a question confidently.

On occasion, the interviewers may ask you to critically appraise a specific paper, which you will be given a reasonable amount of time (anything between 20 and 60 minutes) to read prior to the interview. To perform well, you will obviously have in mind a process to critically appraise a paper; this chapter will also help you considerably with this task.

9.1 Tell us about your teaching experience

This is a fairly straightforward question, where you can easily shine, provided that you give an answer that goes beyond the obvious day-to-day informal teaching experience that you may have. Indeed, most marking schemes allocate very few marks for informal teaching experience and reward candidates who show more initiative and enthusiasm towards teaching. To optimise your marks, you will need to provide as much information as possible in each of the following sections.

Section 1: Actual teaching experience

You can structure this section in two ways:

Structure 1	Structure 2
Different types of teaching	Different types of groups taught

<ul><li>Informal teaching</li><li>Lectures (big groups)</li><li>Workshops</li><li>Presentations
  – Departmental
  – Regional
  – National</li></ul>
	<ul><li>Undergraduate dental students</li><li>Dental care professionals, wider members of the dental team</li><li>Teaching outside dentistry (if you do some)</li></ul>

Whatever structure you choose, you will need to describe the extent of your teaching experience, covering:

- The types of groups you have taught
- The teaching methods you used (e.g. simulation, role play)
- The types of topics that you taught (e.g. clinical knowledge/skills, procedures, history taking, breaking bad news)

Most marking schemes allocate further marks if the candidate has organised teaching sessions and/or written teaching material from scratch (as opposed to simply delivering teaching to a group of people). Therefore, if you have shown initiative in organising teaching groups or in writing your own lectures, make sure that you highlight it clearly.

Describe how you plan your teaching to meet the needs of the learners and how you use questions and answers to monitor their progress and understanding. Do you use any form of MCQ/quiz at the end to assess their learning? Do you evaluate the process of your teaching (i.e. how it went and what you could do to improve)?

Section 2: Teaching courses attended

If you have attended any teaching courses, mention them. They will form part of the marking scheme and will reflect the care that you demonstrate in developing your skills. Do not limit yourself to stating that you attended a course; explain also what you gained from it and how it helped you improve your teaching skills. Remember, the more personal your answer is, the stronger its impact.

Section 3: Feedback

- ### Collecting feedback
  The interviewers will want to know that you take teaching seriously and that you make an effort to find out what others think of your performance. This will portray the image of someone who is keen to improve constantly. In this section, you should therefore explain how you seek feedback from those you teach. Hopefully, this will be through formal means such as a questionnaire being distributed at the end of the teaching session. However, if you have not collected formal feedback, then you can of course talk about how you collect informal feedback from colleagues. Generally speaking, introducing qualitative feedback into your answer (e.g. "The vast majority of the students enjoyed it because ...") will have a better effect than presenting quantitative feedback (e.g. "All of the dental students gave me 9/10").

- ### Nature of the feedback
  As well as explaining that you collect feedback, you can push the answer further, by stating what that feedback is (limiting yourself to the positive feedback). Sell yourself by stating what others think of your teaching (e.g. that you are very organised, very good at expressing complex ideas in simple terms, good at anticipating the audience's needs).

Section 4: Why you enjoy teaching and future plans

The marking schedule will allow for your enthusiasm and commitment. You should therefore emphasise how important teaching is in dentistry and explain what you enjoy about it (see question 9.2 for ideas). If you have specific plans for the future, e.g. taking up a medical/dental education degree or getting involved with British Dental Association or Royal College teaching and training initiatives, then you should mention them. Perhaps you are keen to take up a junior trainee group representative role with an association such as the British Society of Oral Medicine, which will involve organising and/or delivering teaching regionally.

9.2 Why do you enjoy teaching?

There are many things that one can enjoy about teaching, and you will most likely be able to come up with your own reasons. Generally speaking, you may wish to consider the following points:

- You get personal satisfaction from participating in the development of your colleagues, and the feedback you have been getting certainly shows that people appreciate your input.

- It helps the team bond together. By spending time with your colleagues, away from the pressures of your daily routine, you can build better working relationships, which in turn translates into better patient care and a good atmosphere at work (well, sometimes, anyway!).

- You can learn a lot from teaching others. Not only do they force you to know your topic in depth (they might ask all sorts of questions at the end of the session), but you also learn through the preparation that you do. For example, to prepare for a teaching session, you may need to go over your textbooks again, reading journals, looking up guidelines, etc.

Back up each of these points (and any others you may have decided upon) with personal examples. For example, for the third point (learning during the preparation of the teaching session), take the specific example of a recent talk that you prepared and explain what you learnt (or consolidated) as a result.

9.3   What are the qualities of a good teacher?

This is a general question (i.e. not explicitly asking about your own qualities) but, nevertheless, the marking schedule will expect you to go beyond the general approach, to discuss your own skills and experience. We suggest that you answer this question in two sections:

Section 1 – General answer

Describe what makes a good teacher, explaining why each quality is important. To make the answer more interesting, you can draw upon your experience, illustrating your answer by talking about how you were particularly well taught or inspired by a specific consultant or speaker. Here are some of the key qualities of a good teacher:

- Sets appropriate, specific and challenging goals
- Has a clear plan to achieve his/her goal and has a clear delivery of his/her topic
- Involves the students, continually assesses the learning and provides feedback
- Is positive and encouraging
- Is able to promote enthusiasm in his/her students
- Is able to adapt to the students and alter his/her methods accordingly
- Is resourceful and adopts a problem-solving approach
- Respects his/her students
- Gathers feedback and reflects on negative feedback

Section 2 – Personal experience

Explain that these are qualities that you try your best to incorporate into your own teaching. Give one or two examples of situations where you have been able to motivate and enthuse a group of students about a given topic. Mention as a conclusion that you get good feedback from your teaching sessions, and state briefly what people appreciate about your teaching.

9.4 How do you know that you are a good teacher?

Many candidates often rush to list the skills and attributes that make them a good teacher (i.e. basically, they answer the previous question instead: "What are the qualities of a good teacher?"). This question is not about whether you are good, but about how you *know* that you are good. There are many ways in which you may know that you are good, including:

- Positive feedback from colleagues. The feedback could come either from a form that you distribute after each of your sessions, from formal feedback at appraisals (360-degree feedback or MSF – multi-source feedback)

- Being asked to become an instructor on an ALS course (or other similar course)

- Being re-invited to teach at a course (thus indicating that the first time was successful)

- Objective measures of success such as colleagues passing their exams as a result of your teaching

- Visible improvements on the shop floor, for example a junior becoming much more efficient and safer doing a procedure that you taught him/her

- The way in which your students interact with you during teaching sessions, i.e. the interest they pay to the topic

When you deliver your answer, do not simply list some or all of the above. Each time you bring up a point, illustrate it with experience. For example, do not just state that your feedback was positive. Describe what the feedback was (stick to the positive feedback). If you have been re-invited to teach at a course, explain why this was the case. What did they like about you the first time round?

9.5 Which methods of teaching do you know?

This question is not too difficult but, again, the difficulty is in making your answer sound interesting and personal. Most candidates limit themselves to listing a few teaching methods they have come across, without feeling the need to expand. The marking scheme will reward candidates who show an awareness of different teaching methods, their advantages and disadvantages, and who relate their answers to their own personal experiences.

Present a broad spectrum of methods

The question is asking about the teaching methods that you *know*, not just those that you *use*. Make sure that you present not only the methods that you have encountered or used yourself, but also other methods that you may not have come across. For example, some people may know about the existence of virtual learning environments (VLEs) or flipped classroom teaching methodology (preloading with virtually delivered information prior to a face-to-face interaction with a teacher or trainer) but have no direct experience of being on the receiving end of these teaching methods. Technology enhanced learning (TEL) in particular is on the agenda for most organisations involved in the delivery of postgraduate and undergraduate education.

Expand on each method

The interviewers will be looking for awareness and understanding of the different methods. In your answer, you should therefore present not only your own experience of these methods (to the extent that you have any) but also what you know of the pros and cons of each method. No need to go into massive detail – a brief explanation will suffice.

The different teaching methods

There is a wide array of teaching methods. We have set out below those that you may encounter more commonly:

One-to-one interactive teaching
- Pros: you can tailor the teaching to the needs, strengths and weaknesses of the student. It encourages maximum participation from the student and therefore optimises the learning experience. One-to-one teaching also offers flexibility because there is only one person to worry about.

- Cons: It is time-consuming, and the student does not have the opportunity to learn from listening to or watching his/her peers.

Small-group interactive teaching (workshops, tutorials)

- Pros: interaction between different group members can raise the quality of the teaching (i.e. students feed off one another). The teaching can benefit from the experience of the various students rather than just one. It is easy to gauge the mood and understanding of the group and for the teacher to deviate from the prepared material, if there is a need to do so during the session. One particular type of teaching is known as interprofessional learning (IPL). This is defined as learning with, from and about other professionals (e.g. dental hygienists, dental therapists, pharmacists) to improve collaboration in practice and quality of care for the patient (Centre for Advancement of Interprofessional Education – www.caipe.org.uk).

- Cons: if the group is not homogeneous, some members may feel that they are struggling, whilst others may feel that they are not being stretched enough. If you are teaching a group of individuals, it is therefore important that you enquire beforehand about their levels of knowledge and, if possible, that you circulate material so that those who have lesser knowledge are able to raise their game before the teaching session. This is particularly important for IPL, where the students need to be at the same level (e.g. similar clinical exposure if undergraduate) and secure in their professional identities.

Formal (didactic) lectures

- Pros: you can reach a big audience quickly.
- Cons: the communication is mostly one-way. It can be difficult to give everyone in the group what they expect from the lecture. The structure is usually fairly rigid, and there is limited allowance for questions and interaction. It is difficult for the lecturer to gauge the level of understanding of the students, which may result in loss of attention. Many people rely on very poor slide presentations. You can, however, use technology such as polling software, many of which are free to access and use (e.g. www.kahoot.com, as one example among many), but in many institutions the TEL team will have in-house options to offer.

Virtual learning environments / online learning / e-Learning

- Pros: the student can take the modules at his/her own pace and can undertake the teaching at a time when he/she is the most receptive. e-Learning can also enable learning by repetition without boring the teacher. It is also possible to learn at a distance, even internationally.
- Cons: only works if well structured, since the student has no opportunity to address a human being. The exception to this is "flipped" learning, where the online distance-learning component is delivered in advance of a face-to-face teaching event, which aims to consolidate or apply the knowledge gained in a much shorter space of time. Webinars are another great way of bridging this divide and enabling e-Learning to be more interactive. Health Education England have an excellent platform called "e-Den", delivered as part of the e-Learning

for Healthcare (www.e-lfh.org.uk), which is an exemplar of online learning resources. A familiarity with common learning management platforms (e.g. Moodle, Canvas, among others) would be worthwhile here.

Within each of the above settings, there are different ways of delivering teaching such as:

- Interactive discussion
- Practical simulation
- Role play
- Observation followed by repeated practice under assisted supervision and silent supervision (e.g. to learn clinical procedures)
- Problem-based learning (these days increasingly used in undergraduate education: see next question for full details)
- Lecture followed by assessment

9.6 What is problem-based learning (PBL)? What are its pros and cons?

Problem-based learning is a teaching method based on a small group of students (typically 6 to 10), who are working together, with the help of a tutor. The process is best described by the Maastricht "seven jump" process, *BMJ ABC of learning and teaching in medicine: Problem based learning* (2003), as follows:

Step 1	Identify and clarify unfamiliar terms presented in the scenario; the "scribe" lists those that remain unexplained after discussion
Step 2	Define the problem or problems to be discussed; students may have different views on the issues, but all should be considered; scribe records a list of agreed problems
Step 3	"Brainstorming" session to discuss the problem(s), suggesting possible explanations on basis of prior knowledge; students draw on each other's knowledge and identify areas of incomplete knowledge; scribe records all discussion
Step 4	Review steps 2 and 3 and arrange explanations into tentative solutions; scribe organises the explanations and restructures if necessary
Step 5	Formulate learning objectives; group reaches consensus on the learning objectives; tutor ensures learning objectives are focused, achievable, comprehensive, and appropriate
Step 6	Private study (all students gather information related to each learning objective)
Step 7	Group shares results of private study (students identify their learning resources and share their results); tutor checks learning and may assess the group

In PBL, the tutor is a facilitator (and not necessarily a clinician), i.e. he/she does not participate actively in the discussions. He/she is there to motivate and guide the team, helping it define and reach its objectives. This is in stark contrast to the traditional teaching methods, where the teacher has a very active role. In PBL, students are discovering for themselves, under remote supervision and guidance.

Advantages of PBL

- It is a flexible way of learning, doing away with the rigidity of traditional lectures.

- Being self-directed, students think for themselves and discover the information by themselves. This tends to lead to better retention.

- PBL does not simply promote learning the topic. It encourages students to develop other skills such as problem solving (they are confronted by a problem they have never faced before), communication (they need to argue their case to the rest of the team) and teamwork (regardless of personal opinions, it is the team as a whole which needs to resolve the problem).

- PBL allows students to make mistakes and to learn from them (the worst that can happen is wasting time). This may create broader-minded and more adventurous individuals, who can simultaneously adopt a reflective approach and do not hesitate to ask for help.

- PBL promotes initiative, focus on specific goals and research.

- Because the learning is problem-based, PBL is good at helping students place problems in the overall perspective and from a practical point of view. Students are not just learning information that could be useful to them in the future; the scenario actually shows them how the information and knowledge could be used in a concrete situation.

Disadvantages of PBL

- PBL calls for more resources than traditional teaching methods, because the groups cannot be too large.

- The preparation that the tutor needs to undertake can be extensive. For example, he/she may need to prepare extensive reading lists and web-based resources. The tutor may also need to make himself available outside of the normal workshops in case queries arise.

- Many students are not used to PBL and may feel disorientated when confronted with such an unfamiliar method. This can be stressful.

- PBL relies on good teamwork and therefore may not function well in less homogenous groups (e.g. if one of the team does not contribute).

- If not facilitated properly, the group may easily diverge and waste time.

- The information accumulated by students is the result of their research. There is a danger that students retain information which either they do not need to know or which is too advanced for their level.

9.7 You have been asked to organise a weekly educational meeting for your colleagues. How would you approach this task?

Many of the clinicians who have been asked this question and with whom we have talked have found it difficult to answer because they had "never organised a meeting before". In reality, if you think carefully about the skills that are being tested and use your logic, you should be able to provide a complete answer without much of a problem.

What is this question about?

As mentioned, this question is about your organisational skills, i.e. your ability to manage resources, time and information appropriately. It is also about your ability to work with others and communicate appropriately to achieve a positive outcome.

If you have never organised such meetings, think logically about what this would involve. Much of the content can be derived using common sense. Think about the type of meeting that you would like to be invited to:

- What would you like to learn?

- Who would you like to hear from?

- What is your objective? To organise a meeting that people will want to go to (otherwise you are wasting your time).

- It is a weekly meeting. You will need to make sure that your colleagues want to attend every week. To achieve this, you will need to organise events of quality and make participants feel involved. You cannot achieve this without ensuring that you understand what your colleagues are expecting from the educational meetings.

- If it is a weekly meeting, you cannot do all the work by yourself. You will need to arrange for different speakers, and you will need to get the logistics sorted out (booking a room, photocopying the handouts, drinks, maybe sponsorship). All this takes time and you will need to get help from someone.

- You will need to make sure people can attend; therefore, your meeting will need to be at a convenient time.

Much of your success will depend on your ability to communicate and work with others. You should therefore make sure that this is explicit in your answer.

Structuring the answer to the question

There are many ways in which you can structure your answer. Here is a suggestion:

Defining the meeting

- Because it is a weekly meeting, you will need to find new topics every week as well as new presenters. In order to ensure the success of your project and to ensure that your colleagues get as much as they can out of the meetings, you will need to approach them and ask them what type of topics would interest them, when is the most suitable time for them and whether there are topics that they may wish to present themselves. This can be done either face to face or via a simple questionnaire, which they can complete.

- Subjects can include:
  - Topics on the dental core and/or specialty training curriculum
  - Topics defined by available local speakers
  - Topics on the previous timetable
  - Risk management/patient safety
  - Journal club
  - Case of the week
  - Management/leadership
  - Quality improvement

- You will also probably need to involve some of your senior colleagues, who may have their own ideas about what can be achieved through these meetings. They may also have ideas that would make your life easier.

- Once you have gathered some basic information about the type of topics your colleagues want to discuss and what your seniors are aiming for, you can start putting together a document that summarises your findings and that you can discuss with your consultant. The two of you can then settle on a format and an appropriate time.

- You may also wish to discuss with your seniors whether you should limit the meeting to your immediate colleagues, or whether it should be open to other departments, and even other professions (nurses, secretaries, etc), in the team.

Sorting out the practicalities

- Once the meeting has some shape, you will need to ensure that people can attend it. You should probably have a discussion with rota coordinators or personnel involved in staffing clinics so that they can ensure that the time is protected and that all clinical duties are either cancelled or covered appropriately.

- You should also liaise with a secretary, to ensure that the meeting is advertised appropriately, that a room is booked and that all speakers have been notified of their engagement.

- You should be in touch with the speakers regularly, to ensure that they are on track (otherwise you will have no meeting) and to arrange for any material to be given in advance (using the secretary for photocopying).

Running the meeting

- Ensure that the meeting is chaired appropriately, either by you or by someone else.

- Make sure you know how to use the computer and projector (if used), as this can be the easiest way for things to fail.

- Ensure that the session is well paced, so that the meeting is not too rushed or too slow.

- Ensure that those who attend have opportunities to ask questions so that they fully benefit from the meeting.

Learn from the experience and improve

- Collect feedback at the end so that you can improve from one session to the next. Remember to include space for free text:
  - What went well (and why)?
  - What should we do differently next time?

Remember as well that, if you want to develop this in line with General Dental Council verifiable continuing professional development (CPD) requirements under the new enhanced CPD scheme (which would certainly do no harm to attendance rates!), then you will have to satisfy the following requirements are demonstrated and defined:

- The CPD subject, learning content, aims, and objectives
- The anticipated GDC development outcome(s) of the CPD
- The date that the CPD was undertaken
- The total number of hours of CPD undertaken
- The name of the practitioner who participated in the CPD activity
- Confirmation that the CPD provided has been quality assured, including the name of the person or body responsible for completing quality assurance
- Confirmation that the information is complete and accurate
- Inclusion of the participant's registration number

In addition, there should be a defined quality assurance (QA) element to the provision of your educational event, to satisfy the requirements of the GDC. These are defined in the GDC guidance document *Enhanced CPD: Guidance for providers*, which is available online at https://www.gdc-uk.org/docs/default-source/enhanced-cpd-scheme-2018/cpd-provider-guidance.pdf?sfvrsn=63766c6a_2

9.8   Tell us about the feedback that you have received for your teaching

Aim of the question

The aim of the question is not just to see whether you are any good at teaching (the interviewers will need to take your word for it). The question also aims to determine whether you have any insight into your own strengths and weaknesses, and whether you are able to build on the feedback that you receive and improve as a result of action taken.

The question does not explicitly state whether you should limit your answer to the positive feedback or also discuss the negative feedback that you have received. However, the marking scheme will definitely require both to be presented, and you should therefore do so without waiting to be prompted.

Getting the positive–negative balance right

Whenever you face a question asking you for both positive and negative aspects of yourself, you should aim to present slightly more positive points than negative. Here you ought to aim at two or three positive points against one negative point. There are two reasons for this:

- You obviously want to emphasise your strengths more than your weaknesses.

- When talking about the negative feedback, you will need to spend time explaining how you learnt from it. This will take time. Overall, you will find that discussing one weakness will take as much time as discussing two strengths.

The positive points should come first, followed by the negative point. This has the advantage of enabling you to start the answer in an enthusiastic manner, and to conclude it with the reflective part of the negative feedback, which will leave an impression of maturity. Starting with the negative point, without setting out a positive context, will leave a gloomy impression.

Example of an effective answer

"The feedback that I have obtained from colleagues and students has always been very positive and encouraging. One of the points, which people often mention, is that my teaching sessions are well structured and that, as a result, I am able to maintain the audience's attention for long periods of time. Dental students also very much appreciate the attention that I pay to making my sessions interactive. They have found that they retained the information much more and many of them have actually obtained good results in their finals as a result.

"On the less positive side, there was a specific workshop, for which I had not anticipated the diversity of backgrounds of the students and, in particular, I had not taken account of the fact that half of them had already had experience of the specialty, whilst the other half had not. At the time, this caused some problems with comprehension.

"Since this particular incident, I take much greater care to discuss with the students before the session what they know and what they seek to gain from the session, and I have not had any more issues."

This answer is effective because:

- There is a good balance between positive and negative. The two paragraphs are of equal length.

- The negative feedback is well presented, with an element of personal reflection, which emphasises the candidate's willingness to learn.

- The negative feedback is specific and refers to a temporary error of judgement rather than lasting incompetence. It has also been remedied.

Example of an effective answer (partial – negative paragraph only)

"As far as negative feedback is concerned, there have been a couple of occasions where people commented on the fact that my slides were too wordy. It is an issue which I think is quite common and to resolve this I attended a presentation skills course at the Royal College of Surgeons, as a result of which I have learnt to make better use of pictures and diagrams. I have also become more conscious of the fact that you don't need to put everything down on your slides and that it can be just as effective to address the audience directly, with the slide showing just the key headings. It makes the speaker more engaging."

9.9 Tell us about a bad (or your worst) teaching experience that you have had as a teacher (i.e. not as a delegate)

Whether you are asked about a bad or your worst teaching experience makes no difference at all. As always, when asked about something negative, you will be expected to explain how you have dealt with it and how you learnt from it; therefore, what matters more is that you choose an experience that enables you to sell yourself effectively.

Examples you can mention

Since the emphasis is on the reflective process, you should choose an example that has potential for this. This may include situations where:

- Your teaching session was too complicated or too easy for your audience.
- Your audience was made up of people who had very varied backgrounds.
- You had to deal with disruptive students in your audience.
- You failed to prepare adequately (e.g. unable to answer questions).
- One of your audience/group consistently failed to understand what you were trying to teach them and you struggled through multiple alternatives.

Note that you don't have to mention your *actual* worst experience if you really messed up. No one will know what the truth is. Simply choose any negative experience on which you reflected meaningfully.

Structuring your answer

To answer this question, you can follow the STAR structure (see 5.2):

Situation/Task	Explain what type of teaching session it was and why it went wrong
Action	Demonstrate the initiative that you used at the time to correct the problem. How did you communicate? How did you alter your plans to adapt to the changing circumstance?
Result/Reflect	What happened at the end? What did you learn from the situation? How has it helped you improve your teaching abilities?

9.10 What is clinical audit?

With this question, the interviewers will be testing your understanding of the audit process, and you will therefore need to go well beyond giving out a simple definition. They will be expecting you to raise two points:

- A clear explanation of what an audit is, i.e. a definition in your own words
- A description of the audit cycle

Definition of clinical audit

There are several definitions of clinical audit, some of which date back to 1989 and 1983. An excellent and concise definition is that published in *Principles for Best Practice in Clinical Audit* (2002) by the National Institute for Clinical Excellence (NICE) (since renamed the National Institute for Health and Care Excellence):

> "Clinical audit is a quality improvement process that seeks to improve patient care and outcomes through systematic review of care against explicit criteria and the implementation of change. Aspects of the structure, processes and outcomes of care are selected and systematically evaluated against explicit criteria. Where indicated, changes are implemented at an individual, team, or service level and further monitoring is used to confirm improvement in healthcare delivery."

The full document is available at:
https://www.nice.org.uk/media/default/About/what-we-do/Into-practice/principles-for-best-practice-in-clinical-audit.pdf

At an interview, beware of trying to regurgitate definitions. Most are lengthy, use words which are not natural to you, and sometimes are deliberately vague to cover wide areas. Your task is therefore to transform this definition into something more easily digestible. For example:

> "Clinical audit is a review of current health practices against agreed standards, designed to ensure that, as clinicians, we provide the best level of care to our patients and that we constantly seek to improve our practice where it is not matching those standards."

Or

> "Audits are a systematic examination of current practice, to assess how well an institution or a practitioner is performing against set standards. Essentially, it is a method for systematically reflecting on, reviewing and improving practice."

The audit cycle

Some of the marks for this question will relate to your understanding of the audit cycle. Make sure that you can discuss each of the following steps without hesitation:

Step 1: Identify an issue or problem

The aim of an audit is to ensure that your clinical practice is in line with best practice. Dental care professionals should continually audit their practice, in turn identifying and making changes where required. Primary target topics for audits may include:

- Any area of clinical practice where problems have arisen; this could have been identified through a rising level of complaints, the occurrence or recurrence of mistakes
- The need to check compliance with national guidelines
- Areas of clinical practice where there are clear risks, either because they deal with a high volume of patients or because there are high costs associated with these procedures/practices
- Any obvious areas where improvements can be brought in (often identified through observation or experience)

Step 2: Identify a standard

Clinical practice will be assessed against a standard, which needs to be defined at the outset. Standards should be drawn from the best available evidence and in many cases are set by NICE, the faculty of dental surgery/dentistry of one of the royal colleges, or other specialty-related associations (e.g. British Orthodontic Society). When standards are not readily available, an NHS trust or primary dental care provider may define its own local standards. A trust or primary dental care provider may also want to impose on itself standards that are more stringent than those available.

Step 3: Collect data on current practice

The data should be collected in respect of a pre-agreed period of clinical practice (e.g. period between date one and date two), for a specific group of individuals (e.g. all asymptomatic patients who presented to clinic for the first time). These criteria will have been agreed at the outset. In collecting data, care should be taken to ensure that any patient identifiable data is removed.

Note that there are clinical audit departments in organisations such as acute and community trusts, which exist to support your audits! As such, they will help design proformas, collect notes, possibly even do any statistical analysis required, and then help present the data. The important thing is to start early and communicate with them.

Step 4: Assess conformity of clinical practice with the standard

Once the data has been summarised and analysed, the result is compared with the standard, to determine how well it has been met.

More importantly, if the standard is not met, the reasons for non-compliance should be identified so that they can be remedied. Although identifying non-compliance is relatively easy, identifying why there is a problem may take more time. In some cases, it may be necessary to carry out a study of the problem to understand the causes of the underperformance.

Step 5: Implementing change

This is the step that justifies the whole process, i.e. improving practice so that the standard is matched. Examples of changes may include:

- Altering protocols (especially simplifying them)
- Reorganising service, altering roles and responsibilities
- Providing further training to key staff
- Raising awareness of guidelines with staff (e.g. regular teaching sessions, creation of an intranet)
- Improving documentation
- Altering a labelling system
- Changing equipment

Step 6: Closing the loop: re-audit

Once all changes have been implemented, the dust should be allowed to settle. After an agreed period of time, once the changes have had a chance to have an impact on clinical practice, clinical practice should be audited again to measure their impact. To be effective and meaningful, a re-audit should use the same sample, methods and data analysis. Hopefully, the re-audit will show that the standard has been matched. If not, further changes will be required and further re-audits should be carried out.

Carrying out the re-audit is commonly referred to as "closing the loop" or "completing the audit cycle". This is by far the weakest point of the process, partly because of turnover of staff and partly because the process of audit still remains poorly understood.

Note: it may be that, in the meantime, the standard has changed (e.g. in view of new research). In this case, the re-audit will constitute a new audit and it can be referred to as the "audit spiral".

9.11 Tell us about an interesting audit that you did

Structuring your answer

This question is designed to test your understanding of the audit process/cycle, through the description of one example. To demonstrate that you understand clearly the principles of audits, you should therefore aim to address explicitly the following points:

- **Why the audit was deemed necessary** (i.e. what was the problem which led to the initiation of an audit?).

- **The standard used.** Typically, this would be guidelines from a faculty of dental surgery / dentistry of one of the royal colleges or some other association; but it may be that you had to derive your own standard, by doing a literature search, for example. If this is the case, be sure to mention it.

- **The result of the audit,** i.e. did clinical practice match the standard, and if not, why not?

- **What proposals for change you made, and which were implemented**

- **Whether you did a re-audit or not.** If you did not do the re-audit (which will be the case for the vast majority of candidates), make sure that you demonstrate your understanding of this crucial step by saying something such as "Since this was the end of my attachment, I did not have time to be involved in the re-audit, but we planned it for six months down the line". If you have taken the trouble to check the results of the re-audit with the local team, then this would be to your credit, because it would demonstrate the effectiveness of the changes that you had proposed and implemented.

Consider doing a re-audit as your audit. This will save all the planning and thinking and show that you understand the process. Remember that maximum marks are often attributable to closing the loop. Sometimes, all it takes is a phone call to the current incumbent of your old post, to see whether they have re-audited on your project and what their findings were. If they haven't picked up the re-audit of your project yet, they are probably scratching their heads thinking of a suitable audit project and will welcome your call!

- **What your role was** (i.e. initiated, devised a proforma, collected the data, analysed, discussed with senior colleagues, identified ideas for change, wrote report, presented to local team/audit meeting).

- **Presentation/publication.** If the audit was presented outside the local environment, or even published either as such or as an abstract, make sure that you mention it. Remember that good audits are really only locally valuable and rarely yield transferable insights, as they are site-specific and only offer guidance on the way you do things. Audits are standards-driven, as opposed to research, which is hypothesis-driven and truly transferable. That said, there is often value in disseminating findings as, at the very least, it may prompt others to examine their own practice, particularly if your standard was developed from the literature and not freely available.

Choosing an "interesting" audit

The question uses the word "interesting". However, it is possible that the audit that you personally enjoyed the most is not the audit that will score the most points.

Your main criterion for the choice of an example should be the extent of your involvement in the project and the strength/complexity of the audit, as these are the factors that will influence the marking the most. That, and whether or not you closed the loop!

If you can, focus on an audit that is relevant to the specialty to which you are applying. Not only might some marks be allocated for the relevance of the example to the specialty, but, even if this is not the case, the interviewers will be naturally drawn towards an example which they can relate to. Of course, if you find that you have no specialty-related audits that are of any interest but that another audit would make a far more powerful answer then use the latter.

Concluding your answer

The use of the word "interesting" in the question means that you really ought to explain why you feel that the particular audit you have just described is "interesting". It could be because of the topic itself, or because of the potential for change that it offered. It may also be because it gave you an opportunity to develop new skills such as delegation and management, and perhaps IT too. Whatever your reasons, make sure that you explain them (albeit succinctly).

You may also emphasise how much this experience taught you about the audit process and how it gave you an impetus to become involved in other audit projects. You can then name a project in which you are currently involved (name, not describe, otherwise it will take too long).

9.12 Tell us about your audit experience

How this question is marked

The marking schemes for this question vary widely between panels, specialties and grades. Some interview panels will simply assess on the number and quality of the audits that candidates have done, whilst others will use much more complex criteria, even at the most junior levels. Generally speaking, in dental core training and specialty training interviews, it is likely that the number of audits and evidence of clinical governance participation *per* se is examined, with reference to the portfolio as part of a structured scoring system. The clinical governance station then allows more in-depth explanation of your understanding and personal involvement with audit, e.g. in describing an audit you have done and/or are especially proud of.

Across the board then, the interviewers will assess you on the following criteria:

- **The number of audits** in which you have been involved. This will be judged in relation to the expectation at your level. Most DCTs and DFTs are expected to complete one audit per post, or at least two a year.

- **Your role in the audit process.** If you have been involved simply in collecting data, then you are most likely to score less than if you have initiated and/or led an audit. Doing audits with one or two others allows you to complete more in the time, and chop and change roles.

- **The complexity of your audits.** You will need to explain what the audits were about and what standards you were testing clinical practice against. A minor audit will impress less than a complex audit. Not all interview panels allocate marks to complexity, but those that don't still account for it subconsciously, because the answer will sound more impressive if the audits are complex. Any audit that makes a change and is then re-audited will score well, however simple.

- **The usefulness of your audits**, i.e. the extent to which they identified variation from the standard and led to change. There may be extra marks allocated to candidates who have formed evidence-based guidelines as a result of their audits.

- **Whether you understand the audit process/cycle**

- **Whether or not you completed the loop.** This is unlikely to be relevant for most trainees, as many of you will have moved on before you could perform a re-audit. Remember, it's always worth a phone call to the current incumbent of your previous post, and the last occupier of your present post. There have been various attempts to formalise this process of a baton relay of audit completion, such as the Maxillofacial Trainees Research Collaborative (MTReC), which focuses predominantly on junior staff at DCT level.

- **Whether the audit results were presented** and at what level (i.e. just local, or regional, or even national). Some marking schemes provide further marks for abstracts. Remember the caveats regarding transferability given above. Sometimes, the best audits are the least transferable, because they tell you the most about your current practice, something unique to you and your immediate working environment.

In order to prepare for this question, you would therefore be well advised to draw a list of your audits, and to establish for each of them whether you can gain marks in any of the above categories.

Delivering your answer

If you have done more than two audits, you can introduce your overall experience with a sentence of the type:

> "I have carried out five audits over the past four years, including three that I led personally from initiation to conclusion. Two of these audits were extremely useful in improving clinical care."

Or

> "Over the past four years, I have conducted five audits, including three that are specifically related to <specialty that you are applying for>. The most interesting audits were ..."

You would then develop the two audits in question, in line with the marking criteria set out on the previous page and the structure set out in 9.11.

If you have done one or two audits, then you can simply take them one by one, ensuring that you limit yourself to a total time of two minutes. Simply detail your experience using the points described in the previous section.

If you have not completed an audit but you have been partially involved, be honest about it, but do not make a negative judgement on your experience such as

"Unfortunately my audit experience is very poor because I did not have the opportunity to be involved". Not only does this tell the interviewers how they should interpret your lack of experience (i.e. negatively), it also does not present you as a proactive individual who seeks the experience he/she needs. Simply concentrate on the facts, and explain whatever you have been involved with and how this has given you a better understanding of the audit process (see 9.10 for more detail).

If you have done no audit at all, then you probably won't score anything, but you might as well try to gain some credit by explaining your understanding of the audit process, trying to relate it to your own experience (see 9.10), which you might have gained by attending departmental clinical governance meetings or training sessions. At least say you are currently planning one with the clinical audit department and will start next week.

9.13 Why are audits important?

This question is very factual and, unless you have reflected on the audit process by yourself, you will simply need to learn a few lines to make sure that you provide a sensible answer.

Here are some of the key benefits of audit:

- As one of the key pillars of clinical governance, audit ensures that quality of care is maintained at an agreed standard. It enables the identification of problems and, through the audit cycle, ensures that solutions are implemented until the desired standard of care is reached.

- Audit encourages services to make better use of resources and therefore become more efficient.

- The data gathered during the audit process can be used:

  - To inform patients about the standard of care that they receive (following a range of new reforms, including the emphasis on patient choice, providing information to patients has become a key priority)

  - To feed the appraisal and assessment process, which forms a key part of the new revalidation process

  - To demonstrate to your trust, its managers and other authorities that you are working efficiently and providing a quality service; this will encourage them to help you develop the service further

  - To share information with other trusts on local practices and their efficacy in meeting standards and providing quality care

- The audit process is a good exercise to train and develop juniors. In an era where the training of junior clinicians in management is often criticised, audits offer a good platform to learn about service improvement and quality of service provision.

9.14 What are the problems associated with the audit process?

To answer this question well, you may wish to distinguish between problems associated with audits generally and problems associated with audits carried out by trainees.

If you have done one or more audits yourself, you must have identified at least one or two of the problems listed below. In delivering your answer, feel free to use your own audit experience to illustrate your answer, in order to give it a more personal, less didactic, slant.

Problems associated with audit generally

- Audits are most often a local process. Though they are useful at improving local practice, they may not be so transferable to other organisations or even departments. Other organisations may not be able to replicate the same approach and, if similar problems are identified, the resolution methods that worked well in one place may not achieve the same results when applied in a different one.

- Audits are often based on retrospective data (usually patient notes). The data available in the notes was not collected for the specific purpose of the audit. Therefore, there may be discrepancies in the way it was recorded and, in some cases, the data may be missing (recording bias).

- Audits identify that there is a problem or a lack of compliance with a given standard; identifying a solution to the problem identified may not be so easy. Further studies may be required, which can be lengthy.

- Although there are audit departments in most NHS trusts, those who actually carry out the audits are most often the clinicians, who have many other responsibilities and therefore may not focus entirely on the process. They are also often inexperienced in that activity. This may lead to delay in the implementation of change.

- Unless there is a strong departmental policy of rationalisation of the audit process, topics are not always chosen in the order of priority. This may mean that important areas are neglected, whilst clinicians take on audits that are affordable in terms of resources and are less time-consuming.

The following two points are problems associated with the consequences of the audit process (though not specifically about the audit process itself):

- Audits may identify that non-compliance is linked with the underperformance of specific members of the team or the criticism of certain practices. This makes audit a useful tool, but may also lead to the demotivation of parts of the team, if some people feel more targeted than others.

- One of the outcomes of audit is the implementation of change in order to improve standards of care. This change may lead to resistance from some members of the team.

These problems are particularly acute when audits are conducted across boundaries, e.g. inter-specialty care of patients within the dental hospital. It is easy to criticise another team (e.g. their referral letters or clinical notes), but is difficult to change and can in fact inflame the situation. The way to overcome this is to jointly audit the patient's pathway and keep the focus on what is best for the patient.

Problems associated with audits being carried out by trainees

- DCTs and DFTs move on frequently and, if they are around long enough to carry out an audit, they are most likely to leave before a re-audit can be performed. From their own perspective, they are unable to see the impact of the changes that they have helped introduce. From the departmental perspective, it may be more difficult to find someone to do the re-audit (less glamorous, and they would not benefit from the input of the junior who originally carried out the audit).

- In some cases, the audit analysis is either not completed or the recommendations are not taken to implementation stage, thus defeating the whole purpose of the exercise.

- DFTs, DCTs and even STs may not command the respect that consultants and other seniors would have. They may find it more difficult to obtain data or gain support for their audit project.

- DFTs, DCTs and STs tend to choose audit topics that are easier and take shorter periods of time. These topics may not be aligned with departmental strategy or may not be of great importance in the overall scale of things (i.e. the audit is a box-ticking exercise to look good on the CV).

9.15 What is the difference between audit and research?

This is a question that most candidates have heard about, and the interviewers know it. There is therefore no excuse for being unprepared. If you have been involved in audit and research activities, then you will be able to draw upon your experience to illustrate your answers.

The fundamental difference

The term "audit" is often confused by clinicians, who describe as "audits" projects that are actually research projects. This is fairly common on CVs and application forms, which is why they are keen to test your understanding at the interview. Your application form and CV will be reviewed at the portfolio station. There is nothing more embarrassing than to describe perfectly the difference between audit and research, only to discover that your own documents contradict your words.

Audit is a process that compares clinical practice against set standards, i.e. you are simply trying to determine whether your practice matches the level of care expected of you. Are you following the established guidelines or your own guidelines? Are you aligned with best practice? How much variability is there within your care processes? Are you a learning organisation? Are you doing what you think you are doing?

Research does not check whether you are complying with standards. Instead, its aim is to create new knowledge, which can then be used to develop new standards of care. Research determines whether new treatments work and to what extent they do. It is also used to determine which treatments are better than others so that appropriate recommendations can be made.

So, essentially, research helps establish best practice, whilst audit checks that best practice is being applied in practice.

Examples

If you are trying to establish any of the following, then this is an audit, because you are trying to establish that your current practice is in line with what would be expected:

- Whether x, y and z are correctly recorded in patients' notes
- Whether test X is being offered to a specific type of patients
- That the complication rate for a specific procedure is less or equal to the percentage specified in the XYZ Association guidelines

If, on the other hand, you are trying to establish any of the following points, then it is research, because you are trying to discover new information, which may then be used to implement new guidelines:

- Whether procedure A gives better outcomes than procedure B
- Whether sending patients advance information improves the take-up rate of a specific procedure
- Whether systematic hand washing decreases infection rate

Other differences

- Research is based on a hypothesis, whereas audit measures compliance against standards.

- Research is theory-driven and a one-off process. Audit is practice-driven and a continuous process.

- Results from research can be generalised. Audit results are mostly relevant locally.

- Research is not always conducted by those involved in service provision. Audits most often are.

- Research may involve experimentation, whereas audits never involve experimentation. Audits are mostly a data-gathering exercise.

- Research may involve trying out new treatments, whereas audits never involve new treatments or interference with the management of the patient.

- Research involves strict selection of candidates, allocating these candidates between different treatment groups and validating sample size. In audit, the sample of patients used is not put together scientifically, sample size is not validated and patients are never placed into different treatment groups.

- Research requires ethical approval. Audits rarely do (ethical issues in audit mainly revolve around confidentiality or collection of that data).

Many audits morph into pseudo-research, where lots of data is collected and a new proforma is designed, but in such cases there is no gold standard, no change to the service and often no uptake or spread within the department (particularly after the enthusiast has left).

9.16   Tell us about your research experience

This question can be asked in all specialties and at all grades, even at grades where many candidates are unlikely to have had any substantial involvement in research. There are easy ways to score points, even if your experience is limited.

The boxes you need to tick

Though the question asks for your experience and nothing more specific, most marking schedules will in fact include much more than that. Again, in DCT and ST interviews, marking of the breadth of your involvement may be done against your portfolio, whilst the clinical governance station forms the mainstay of focus into the *quality* of your involvement and of your understanding. In order to provide an answer that is as complete as possible, you will need to address the following points:

- The number, type and quality of research projects undertaken
- The outcomes of projects, including publications and presentations
- Your role, including any experience of recruiting patients, seeking ethical approval or grant applications
- Research-related skills that you gained from your experience, e.g. literature review, critical appraisal, statistics and general understanding of research principles
- General skills gained from your experience, e.g. writing skills, negotiation, communication, teamwork, planning, time management
- Any relevant courses attended such as research methodology, critical appraisal or statistics courses
- Your future plans with regard to research

Answering the question

- *If you have substantial research experience*, you will not have the time to describe all of it. You should aim to summarise the extent of your experience first, e.g. "I have been involved in four research projects, including one randomised controlled trial, two studies and one national trial over the past four years as part of the PhD that I am currently completing". You could then summarise one or two of your projects (those you are most proud of) before discussing the extent of your publications and presentations. End the answer by mentioning the courses that you attended and discussing your future research aims and interests.

- *If you have been involved in a small number of research projects*, describe each project briefly, setting out your role, the courses you attended, the publications and presentations that originated from your experience and the skills that you gained, as well as your future research aims and interests.

- **If you have no research experience at all**, think carefully first about any project in which you have been involved and which is <u>not</u> an audit. Can this project be considered research, even if it was informal? If yes, then you can present whatever you did in line with the principles explained so far. If not, then don't panic. Many people will be in your situation and you can still score marks by mentioning some of the following:

  - <u>Literature reviews</u> undertaken (which gave you an insight into research principles)

  - <u>Case reports published</u>. Strictly-speaking, case reports do not constitute research, because they are simply reporting how a specific patient presented or was managed. However, by sharing your experience with others, you are helping them change or improve their practice. Other benefits include the literature search you will have completed, the rigour of having to write concisely and the overall experience of how to construct a paper and bibliography. Case reports are part of the <u>pool of evidence</u> used in <u>evidence-based medicine</u> and therefore they are relevant to the "spirit" of the question. Some marking schemes make specific allowance for case reports, so make sure you mention yours

  - Attendance at <u>journal clubs</u> (which will have given you <u>critical appraisal skills</u> and an understanding of the research process)

  - Attendance at <u>conferences</u> (where you have gained an appreciation of <u>research methodologies</u>)

  - <u>Research-related courses</u>

9.17 Why is research important?

Fundamental importance of research – the overall perspective

Essentially, the aim of research is to drive medical/dental advancement by developing a pool of knowledge, which can then be translated into better patient care. Research can therefore benefit patients directly, through improved treatments and procedures. Translation of the key messages from the literature to routine medical/dental practice is, however, very slow.

Importance of research to a trust

- The trust's reputation may be enhanced. Not only might this attract more patients (and therefore more income), but also higher-quality staff and more trainees.

- A trust involved in research through clinical trials can provide some of its patients with early access to the latest technologies for diagnosing and treating disease.

Importance of research to a dentist

- It enables them to understand the evidence on which decisions are based. In particular, the treatments and procedures they are using in their everyday practice would have greater meaning to them.

- Nurturing a practice founded on evidence-based dentistry (EBD – see 9.20) involves an ability to critically appraise current evidence. Having an insight into what constitutes good and bad research, as well as the structure of levels of evidence and statistical concepts, is an excellent basis to develop EBD for the future. This can be gained by undertaking research or even, more simply, by attending journal clubs.

- Since dentistry is constantly evolving, it is essential to keep up to date with current published research. This is one component of continuous professional development (CPD), as mandated by the General Dental Council.

- A good grounding and insight into the ethics and procedures of research is important. Academic trainees, in particular, will have future roles in experimental therapies, development of technologies, or managing patients who may be involved in clinical trials.

- Advances in dentistry are inextricably linked to research, and giving trainees inspiration at an early stage may encourage further advancements in the future.

- It provides a good insight into a specialty and often leads to career progression within that field, even if that had not been the previous intention.

- It enables them to gain a range of skills such as organisational skills (working to deadlines, organising data, planning a project, notation, integrity, etc) and writing and presentation skills.

Delivering the answer

If you have been involved in research, make sure that you illustrate the above points with some of your experience. If you have limited experience of research, then you can simply hold an intelligent discussion using some of the above points.

9.18 Do you think that all trainees should do research?

Interpreting the question

This question is often misunderstood. Many candidates say, "Yes, everyone should do research because research is important". There is no doubt that research is important, but it does not mean that everyone *has* to be involved in it. In popular specialties, research is often done to develop a competitive advantage over peers. This is again a poor reason for doing it.

With this question, the interviewers are testing:
- Your understanding of the pros and cons of undertaking research at a junior level
- Your appreciation of the importance of research to a dentist (which we have addressed in 9.17)

Key points:

- If "research" means time out being taken to undertake a PhD, DDS, MPhil, or other degree, then it is probably not necessary for all trainees to become involved. The reasons for this are that:

    - A lot of research achieves little and/or does not get published.
    - Many research projects do not get completed, due lack of time or lack of funding.
    - The limited funding and resources are best saved for those with real enthusiasm or ability.
    - Some trainees may not particularly like research. Making such a big commitment might demotivate them and be counterproductive.
    - Taking time out to do research means moving away from clinical duties and therefore creating greater difficulties in continuing clinical training. If the research period is too great, there is a danger of deskilling.
    - Formal research is probably best left to those who enjoy it and feel that they can fruitfully contribute, hence the development of an academic training pathway with positions such as academic DFTs, academic clinical fellows, clinical lecturers, senior clinical lecturers, readers and professors. The system therefore recognises that not everyone needs to have a formal research interest.

- Even if they are not formally involved in research, trainees need to understand the principles of research, in order to be safe and effective clinicians. In the context of evidence-based practice, trainees will need to understand how research is conducted, and what makes bad and good research. They will need to be able to critically analyse papers in order to determine their validity and how the findings can be interpreted to help clinical decision making (for more details, see 9.17 – paragraph on the importance of research to dentists). Although first-hand research experience would be useful to gain such understanding, it can also be gained through other means, such as:

- Attending journal clubs
- Attending conferences and relevant courses (statistics, critical appraisal, research methodologies)
- Getting involved in smaller, ad hoc or informal research projects (e.g. one afternoon per week), which will not distract from clinical training
- Doing literature searches, for example to set a standard for an audit or as part of evidence-based practice

Answering the question

In answering this question, it is important that you debate the issue rather than rush into giving a strong opinion. There is no harm at all in having a strong opinion, but you need to ensure that it is put into perspective. You should demonstrate your understanding of research, its importance to clinicians, and the issues raised by introducing research in the training curriculum.

If you have any meaningful experience of research, then make sure that you talk about it in your answer. Rather than discussing the usefulness of research to a trainee from a general perspective, you will gain marks for relating your arguments to your own experience (i.e. discussing how you benefited from your own research experience).

Similarly, if you have little research experience, but feel that you have gained appropriate competencies through other means, then you should state this, confidently.

Your experience is more valuable than any general statement.

9.19 What do you understand by the term "research governance"?

Whenever you hear the word "governance", it refers to a set of rules that govern the way a particular activity should be undertaken. For example, clinical governance sets out the principles that clinicians should follow, to provide the best clinical care for their patients and continuous quality improvement.

"Research governance" is a framework of standards of good practice, applied to research. The full extent of these principles and regulations is set out in a document published by the Department of Health: *Research Governance Framework for Health and Social Care.*[6] This has subsequently been replaced by the *UK Policy Framework for Health and Social Care Research.*[7]

Principles

Key principles are outlined, which apply to health- and social-care research:

1. Safety: That the safety and wellbeing of the individual prevails over the interests of science and society

2. Competence: That people involved in managing and conducting research are appropriately trained

3. Scientific and ethical conduct: That research principles are scientifically sound and guided by ethical principles

4. Patient, service user and public involvement: That patients and service users are involved in the design, conduct and dissemination of research

5. Integrity, quality and transparency

6. Protocol: That the design and protocol are clearly described and justified

7. Legality: That all relevant legislation is given due care and attention

8. Benefits and risks: That anticipated benefits and risks are made clear to participants and benefits are weighed against foreseeable risks

9. Approval: That the research is approved by a research ethics committee and any other required body

---

[6] https://www.gov.uk/government/publications/research-governance-framework-for-health-and-social-care-second-edition

[7] https://www.hra.nhs.uk/planning-and-improving-research/policies-standards-legislation/uk-policy-framework-health-social-care-research/

10. Information: That publicly available information is available on any research conducted (unless precluded and agreed by the relevant ethics committee)

11. Accessible findings

12. Choice: That the autonomy and choice of participants is given due respect and attention

13. Insurance and indemnity

14. Respect for privacy

15. Compliance: That all sanctions are enforced for non-compliance with these principles

16. Justified intervention: That, in the case of interventional research, the body of evidence to date supports deviating from standard treatment

17. Ongoing provision of treatment: That special arrangements are made clear regarding ongoing care following the conclusion of the study period

18. Integrity of the care record

19. Duty of care

9.20   What is "evidence-based dentistry"?

Definition of evidence-based dentistry

Evidence-based dentistry (EBD) has been defined as "the conscientious, explicit, and judicious use of current best evidence in making decisions about the care of individual patients. The practice of evidence-based dentistry means integrating individual clinical expertise with the best available external clinical evidence from systematic research".[8]

In 2000, David Sackett revised his definition as follows: "integration of best research evidence with clinical expertise and patient values."[9] More recently, evidence-based dentistry (EBD) has been defined as "practice that integrates evidence, clinical experience and patient preference".[10] The American Dental Association is often quoted in regard to EBD as a concept, and have defined EBD as "an approach to oral health care that requires judicious integration of systematic assessments of clinically relevant scientific evidence, relating to the patient's oral and medical condition and history, together with the dentist's clinical expertise and the patient's treatment needs and preferences.[11]

The three main pillars

There are three main pillars given in the ADA definition:

1. Dentists' clinical expertise: encompassing diagnostic skills, technical skills and communication skills, to optimise patient management and successful outcomes

2. Patients' needs and preferences: the recognition that there is no textbook right answer for everyone and that considerations such as costs and patients' feelings about more or less invasive treatments need to come into play

3. Relevant scientific evidence: which ideally comes from high-quality research to establish the best practice guidelines, referred to in weighing up the implications of the variable other two pillars

---

[8] Sackett DL, Rosenberg WMC, Muir Gray JA, et al. Evidence-based medicine: what it is and what it isn't. *BMJ* 1996;312:71-72

[9] Sackett DL, et al (2002). *Evidence-Based Medicine: How to Practice and Teach EBM.* Churchill Livingstone, New York

[10] Iqbal A, Glenny AM. General dental practitioners' knowledge of and attitudes towards evidence-based practice. *BDJ* 2002;192;587-591

[11] https://ebd.ada.org/en/about

Five key skills

- The ability to formulate clinical problems into four-part questions with reference to different management options: the patient/problem (P), the intervention (I), the comparison (C) and the outcomes (O), or "PICO", for short

- An efficient electronic search for available evidence of an appropriate type and level

- The ability to appraise that evidence in a meaningful way

- Applying the knowledge to patient care with consideration to preferences, values and circumstances of the case at hand

- Self-evaluation and an evaluation of the process

Answering the question

Step 1: Define briefly what EBD is

You should be wary of using ready-made definitions (the same applies to the classic definition of clinical governance), as they simply demonstrate your ability to regurgitate ready-made answers and do not highlight any personal understanding of the underlying issues.

The above definitions also use words that are unfamiliar to many people and that are best avoided (for example, people may not know that "judicious" means "based on sound judgement").

Try to build your own practical definition, showing that you have a good understanding of what EBD entails. As highlighted above, EBD is essentially a combination of the best available research evidence with your own clinical expertise and judgement. This is then applied to a specific case, taking into account patient values.

Step 2: Explain the different skills involved

Step 3: If you have one, give a brief example of a situation where you used evidence-based dentistry

This might include:

- Having had to deal with a patient for whom normal guidelines did not fit, e.g. we take our management cues on medication-related osteonecrosis of the jaws (MRONJ) from the American Association of Oral and Maxillofacial Surgeons (AAOMS) 2014 position paper, but this is not a panacea, and often, emerging evidence regarding treatment modalities, coupled with unique situations, tests the limits of these guidelines.

- A situation where the existing guidelines were out of date and where you needed to derive your own approach using more recent evidence.

- A situation where national guidelines were not suitable for the local pattern of disease.

- Situations where there are new, controversial treatments, which are not yet in routine practice. You would then evaluate the evidence with your colleagues to devise a local strategy.

- Situations where a patient may have read about a treatment modality in the press and may have a particular interpretation. You would need to review the evidence before presenting your personal or departmental perspective.

- Situations where you have to guide the patient to make an informed decision. This would involve presenting the relevant evidence and the efficacy, benefits and risks of the different options according to the literature.

9.21 What are the different levels of evidence available?

There are three different ways to describe the levels of evidence. The easiest classification system is:

Level	Description
Ia	Systematic review or meta-analysis of randomised controlled trials
Ib	At least one randomised controlled trial
IIa	At least one well-designed controlled study without randomisation
IIb	At least one well-designed quasi-experimental study, such as a cohort study
III	Well-designed, non-experimental descriptive studies, such as comparative studies, correlation studies, case-control studies and case series
IV	Expert committee reports, opinions and/or clinical experience of respected authorities

In our experience, many candidates have learnt the above table and know it well. We would therefore encourage you to try to remember it if you can. If you struggle to remember this, particularly at interview, don't panic. It is important you remain confident and explain what you can.

A simple answer such as: "I cannot remember the exact detail of each level; however, I do know that the different levels of evidence range from the strongest level, which is a systematic review, all the way to the weakest, which is represented by the opinion of experts", may not sound much but it is better than waffling desperately through a confused list.

9.22 In evidence-based dentistry, why does a clinician need to take account of his/her own clinical expertise?

This is a question that is often asked as a follow-up, to test the candidates' understanding of the fundamentals of evidence-based practice.

David Sackett states[12]:

"External evidence can inform, but never replace, individual clinical expertise. [This] expertise will assist the practitioner in deciding whether the external evidence applies to the individual client at all, and, if so, how it should be integrated into the clinical decision."

There are several reasons why evidence alone is insufficient and clinical experience matters. Here are a few:

• The study or trial that constitutes the best available evidence may not be directly relevant to the patient and may need to be adapted. For example, the patient may be in a different age range or ethnicity from those used in the study.

• There may be evidence that the administration of a given treatment has a positive impact on some patients. Judgement is needed to determine whether, for this particular patient, the benefits outweigh the risks.

• The patient may have comorbidities, which may influence the decision.

---

[12] Sackett DL, et al (2002). Evidence-Based Medicine: How to Practice and Teach EBM. Churchill Livingstone, New York

9.23 Is evidence-based dentistry relevant to all dental specialties?

The answer to this question is that evidence-based dentistry is applicable to all dental specialties, but to varying degrees. The reasons are as follows:

- **Different levels of research activities**
  Some dental specialties are very strong on research (either because there is more of a research culture or because research can more easily be carried out due to the sheer number and the homogeneity of the patients the specialty deals with). These specialties therefore have a greater body of evidence than others. In areas where research is lacking, the clinician needs to rely principally on his/her judgement to make a decision.

- **Lack of high-level evidence available**
  In some dental specialties, it may be difficult to find high-level evidence. By itself, this is not a problem, since the clinician would then look for lower levels of evidence. However, such evidence may not be widely published.

- **Individuality of patient**
  The impact of social and environmental factors may be so strong that each decision should very much be taken at an individual level, and no evidence (which is likely to be anecdotal) could be reliably used to make decisions.

- **Little historic information on older treatments**
  Some of the long-standing treatments may not be backed up by much evidence, despite the fact that they are deemed to be effective. This may make it more difficult to compare their efficacy in relation to other treatments.

Answering the question

If you have an example or two (preferably from the dental specialty you are applying for), then use them to illustrate your answer.

9.24 Can you describe what clinical governance is?

A well-known definition that you should avoid

The most widely used definition of clinical governance is as follows:

> "A framework through which NHS organisations are accountable for continually improving the quality of their services and safeguarding high standards of care by creating an environment in which excellence in clinical care will flourish." [13]

Although you should of course familiarise yourself with this definition, there is no need to memorise it. Under pressure, most candidates remember the beginning and the end, and mess up the middle part. Even if you remembered it perfectly, you would only demonstrate that you have a good memory and not that you understand the concept. Instead, you should derive your own practical and down-to-earth definition.

How can you define clinical governance?

Anything that avoids the word "flourish" and can be delivered in your own natural words will do, providing it addresses the concepts of quality and accountability. Here are some examples:

> Clinical governance is a quality assurance process, designed to ensure that standards of care are maintained and improved, and that the NHS is accountable to the public.

> Clinical governance is an umbrella term that encompasses a range of activities, in which clinicians should become involved in order to maintain and improve the quality of the care they provide to patients and to ensure full accountability of the system to patients.

The 7 pillars of clinical governance

Traditionally, clinical governance has been described using 7 key pillars. Although it has been refined over the past few years, this approach remains the easiest to

---

[13] G Scally and L J Donaldson, Clinical governance and the drive for quality improvement in the new NHS in England, *BMJ* (4 July 1998): 61–65

remember and to describe at a trainee interview level. It is also the approach that your interviewers are most likely to expect from you since this is what they would have learnt too. The 7 pillars are as follows:

Clinical effectiveness and research

Clinical effectiveness means ensuring that everything you do is designed to provide the best outcomes for patients, i.e. that you do "the right thing to the right person at the right time in the right place". In practice, it means:

- Adopting an evidence-based approach in the management of patients
- Changing your practice: developing new protocols or guidelines, based on experience and evidence if current practice is shown to be inadequate
- Implementing NICE guidelines, National Service Frameworks and other national standards to ensure optimal care (when they are not superseded by more recent and more effective treatments)
- Conducting research to develop the body of evidence available and therefore enhancing the level of care provided to patients in future

Audit

See 9.10 for full details on clinical audit. The aim of the audit process is to ensure that clinical practice is continuously monitored and that deficiencies in relation to set standards of care are remedied.

Risk management

Risk management involves having robust systems in place, to understand, monitor and minimise the risks to patients and staff, and to learn from mistakes and near misses. When things go wrong in the delivery of care, clinical staff should feel safe admitting it and be able to learn and share what they have learnt. This includes:

- Complying with protocols (hand washing, discarding sharps, identifying patients correctly, etc)
- Learning from mistakes and near misses (informally for small issues, formally for the bigger events – see next point)
- Reporting any significant adverse events via critical incident forms, looking closely at complaints, etc
- Assessing the risks identified by likelihood of recurrence and the severity of impact if an incident did occur; implementing processes to reduce the risk and its impact (the level of implementation will often depend on the budget available and the seriousness of the risk)
- Promoting a blame-free culture, to encourage everyone to report problems and mistakes

Education and training

Dental knowledge and technology continues to evolve and ch
and so education and training are essential for clinicians to ke
professional development needs to be driven by self-directe.
practice, for dentists this involves:

- Attending courses and conferences
- Ensuring that GDC CPD requirements are satisfied with regard to the updated GDC Enhanced CPD Scheme published in 2018 which includes the need
  - To have a personal development plan (PDP)
  - To spread CPD across a five-year CPD cycle
  - To align CPD activity with a GDC development or learning outcome(s)
  - To plan CPD relevant to your particular sphere of practice
- Taking relevant exams
- Regular workplace-based assessment in training, designed to ensure that dentists have the appropriate competencies

Patient and public involvement (PPI)

PPI ensures that the services provided are effective, that improvements are made from the patient's perspective, and that patients and the public are involved in the development of services and the monitoring of treatment outcomes. This is being implemented through a number of initiatives and organisations, including:

- Local patient feedback questionnaires
- The Patient Advice and Liaison Service (PALS) – resolves patient concerns
- National patient surveys organised by the Healthcare Commission, which then feed into trusts' rankings
- Local involvement networks (LINks), which have been introduced to enable communities to influence healthcare services at a local level (these used to be called "patient forums")
- The foundation trust board of governors, elected by members of the local community; it has a say on who runs a hospital and how it should be run, including the services it can provide

Using information and IT

This aspect of clinical governance ensures that:
- Patient data is accurate and up to date.
- Confidentiality of patient data is respected.
- Data is increasingly used to measure the quality of outcomes (e.g. through audits) and to develop services tailored to local needs.

fing and staff management

s relates to the need for:

- Appropriate recruitment and management of staff
- Ensuring that underperformance is identified and addressed
- Encouraging staff retention by motivating and developing staff
- Providing good working conditions

> From the above explanations, you may have noted that some of the pillars are more directly related to the day-to-day responsibilities of a dentist:
>
> - **C**linical effectiveness
> - **A**udit
> - **R**isk management
> - **E**ducation and training
>
> Whenever you discuss clinical governance in an answer, you may prefer to discuss these in more depth and simply mention the other three. You can remember these four key pillars with the mnemonic CARE.

Mnemonics

If you are the type of person who likes to remember information through the use of mnemonics, here are a couple which will enable you to remember all the components of clinical governance:

Patient and Public involvement	**S**taff management
Information and IT	**P**atient and Public involvement
Risk management	**A**udit and IT
Audit	**R**isk management
Training/education	**E**ffectiveness (clinical)
Effectiveness (clinical)	**I**nformation and IT
Staff management	**T**raining/education

208

Answering the question

When asked to talk generically about clinical governance, a good structure for your answer would be as follows:

- Give a brief definition of clinical governance, in your own words
- State and define the four CARE pillars
- List the other three pillars (with brief explanations, if you have time)
- Give brief examples where you have practised clinical governance

Alternatively, you could bring examples within each of the four CARE pillars, instead of bringing them in at the end of the answer. Whatever you do, do not attempt to describe each of the pillars in detail. Discussing an introduction to clinical governance and 7 pillars in two minutes would allocate only 15 seconds per section. Not only are you unlikely to remember everything in the right order, but you will also find yourself speeding through your answer. It is better to talk knowledgeably and confidently about four pillars than to waffle about all 7.

9.25 What is your experience of clinical governance?

Be careful with questions on clinical governance, because it is easy to regurgitate its definition and the 7 pillars without really answering the question. This question does not ask for a description of clinical governance, but for your own experience of it. The examiners will judge you on your overall understanding of governance, and the relevance and clarity of your examples. In order to achieve this, you must choose the pillars that are the most relevant for you, i.e. those that you are most likely to have had experience of. These would typically be the CARE pillars (see previous question).

Here are some questions that will help you think about your experience in each area of clinical governance:

Clinical effectiveness

Have you:
- Played a role in implementing new guidelines or protocols in your department?
- Played a role in facilitating the use of guidelines in your department, for example by creating proformas or checklists?
- Initiated a change to an established protocol because you felt that it was inappropriate?
- Collated a set of guidelines (whether in hard copy or online)?
- Needed to do a literature search or read up on guidelines, to determine the best care for a patient?
- Got any research experience?
- Published case reports or papers?

Audit

Have you:
- Participated in an audit?
- Had opportunities to improve clinical practice with one of your audits?
- Supervised others doing audits?
- Completed an audit, including making changes and re-auditing?

Risk management

Do you:
- Double-check that you are doing the right thing (labels, dosages, etc)?
- Seek help or advice from others appropriately?

- Encourage your juniors to come to see you if they have problems or if they have made mistakes?
- Show support towards juniors (rather than blame them) when they get things wrong? When this happens, do you consider how the system can be improved to ensure that mistakes do not happen again?
- Know what root cause analysis is? This is a thorough investigation into the background surrounding a serious untoward event (critical incident), examining protocols, actions, personnel. One technique is the Five Whys: Why did that happen? And why did that happen? Etc.

Have you:
- Identified a problem with some aspects of care in your team and raised the issue with seniors (i.e. a protocol out of date, a common practice that is not wholly appropriate)?
- Reported any significant issues or near misses?
- Made a mistake or had a near miss that you then reported and discussed with colleagues (or maybe formally recorded through a critical incident form)?
- Dealt with a patient's complaint and ensured that practice changed as a result?

Education and training

Do you:
- Have a personal development plan?
- Attend courses on a regular basis?
- Identify your weak areas and find ways of improving your skills?
- Read about cases you have seen, when you get back from work?
- Observe senior colleagues to learn from their practice?
- Ensure that you teach and train junior colleagues when the opportunity arises (and take the initiative to do so without being asked)?
- Read journals regularly?

Patient and public involvement

Have you:
- Done an audit of patient satisfaction?
- Designed a questionnaire to obtain patient feedback?
- Sought informal feedback from patients on your/your department's performance?
- Been involved in responding to patient concerns about your service?
- Involved patients in the design of either a service or some teaching?

Using information and IT

Do you:
- Anonymise data when you use it for audit or other purposes?
- Correct patient records when they are found to be inaccurate?

Have you:
- Queried data to identify trends and subsequently suggested changes to practice (maybe as part of an audit project)?
- Gained IT skills relating to data handling (e.g. databases, web)?

Staffing and staff management

Have you:
- Had to discuss performance issues with a colleague or had to report underperformance to senior colleagues?
- Taken steps to improve working relationships within a team in which you worked?
- Developed ways of improving relationships with other teams (e.g. nurses, other departments)?
- Made efforts to involve others in projects, when you felt they would benefit from such an involvement?

Delivering your answer

Once you have identified the extent of your experience, all you need to do is list each of your experiences, using the pillars as your structure. For each experience, explain how this contributed towards governance and helped maintain or improve standards of care.

9.26 In your trust, who is responsible for clinical governance?

This question is becoming more and more common, and usually comes as a probing question to a more substantial question on governance.

There are two levels of responsibility that you need to discuss:

- The legal responsibility
- The practical responsibility

Legal responsibility

Since 1999, it is the trust board that is responsible for the quality of care provided by the trust. This is relevant for trusts that manage dental hospitals, as much as it is for acute hospital trusts. That responsibility is exercised through the implementation of clinical governance. As head of the trust board, the chief executive of the trust is ultimately the person who is accountable. Every year, each trust must prepare an annual review of clinical governance. This summarises the quality of care and the implementation of good clinical governance.

Practical responsibility

Although the chief executive and the trust board are responsible, they obviously cannot do all the work by themselves. Their role is therefore to make sure that there are structures in place to ensure that clinical governance is fully embedded at all levels. The responsibility for clinical governance is delegated to the medical director, the nursing director, clinical directors, consultants and, ultimately, all staff. Ultimately, everyone in the organisation is responsible for ensuring that standards of care are constantly maintained and improved.

Answering the question

When you answer the question, discuss the two levels of responsibility. Make sure that you include your own role in implementing clinical governance, using examples.

9.27 What is the difference between a standard, a guideline and a protocol?

This is another common question, which interviewers sometimes narrow down to the difference between a protocol and a guideline.

A standard is a defined level of quality that must be achieved. Standards are used to ensure that quality of care is maintained at the best possible level. Through the process of clinical audit, clinicians compare their own practice to the standards set by NICE, royal colleges or other associations and make appropriate adjustments to their practice, to ensure that any underperformance that has been identified is remedied. Targets are also standards. For example, "By December 2004, all patients requiring emergency admission via the emergency department are admitted to a bed in the hospital, within four hours of arrival." A good example of a comprehensive review is *Standards in Dentistry*, published by the Faculty of General Dental Practitioners.[14]

A guideline is a statement that is designed to assist clinicians in making decisions. Guidelines are recommendations for clinical practice, based on evidence and the local infrastructure. They must be interpreted in the light of the particular patient and settings, as well as the strength of the evidence on which they are based. A good example would be the guideline *Antimicrobial Prescribing for General Dental Practitioners*, published by the Faculty of General Dental Practitioners.[15]

A protocol is a step-by-step approach to dealing with an issue such as managing a patient, checking that the right patient/side is being operated on, dealing with a complaint, etc. Protocols must normally be followed exactly (unlike guidelines, which are subject to interpretation). Their purpose is to ensure that there is a systematic approach to dealing with important issues. These specify diagnostic criteria, investigations for diagnosis and monitoring (what and when), and treatment of the disease and any complications (again, what and when). The minimum dataset for orthognathic surgery, published jointly by the British Association of Oral and Maxillofacial Surgeons and the British Orthodontic Society, is a good example of a rigid protocol of pre- and post-operative requirements for assessment of patients that may/should be adopted by units.

When you answer this question, give examples of each type, based on your practice. As much as possible, choose examples from the specialty to which you are applying (if you don't, they will most likely ask you to quote some, so be prepared).

---

[14] https://www.fgdp.org.uk/SiD/title-page
[15] https://www.fgdp.org.uk/antimicrobial-prescribing-standards/title-page

9.28 How do you critically analyse a paper?

What is critical analysis?

The purpose of evidence-based dentistry is to determine how a patient should be managed, based on best available evidence, the clinician's own clinical judgement and patient values (see 9.20). To determine what constitutes best evidence, it is essential to understand the papers that are published, the value they add to the pool of evidence, the flaws they present, their validity, and their applicability to your patient. The critical appraisal process (i.e. the systematic analysis of a paper) is designed to enable clinicians to draw appropriate conclusions about the usefulness and validity of the published evidence.

How does critical analysis feature at interviews?

At the interview you may simply be asked how you would critically analyse a paper. You may also be asked to critically appraise a real paper. Currently, this features in the National Institute for Health Research (NIHR) academic clinical fellowship (dental) recruitment interviews. In such cases, you will be asked to come early in the day and will be given time to prepare. In this instance you are given a generic dataset/publication to consider for 10 minutes, immediately prior to being interviewed. Scoring domains include the ability to explain the finding to both a scientific and a lay audience. Once you have presented your critical appraisal of the paper, the interviewers may ask questions on the paper itself and the issues it raises. You may also be asked questions on the different types of research and on statistics.

Everyone has their own technique to critically appraise papers, the easiest approach being to go through each section from top to bottom, addressing relevant points as you go. The Faculty of General Dental Practitioners has published a critical appraisal guide.[16] Whichever process you follow, your aim will be to address the key issues, which are set out below:

General background

Title
- Is the title relevant in relation to the content?

Journal
- Is it peer-reviewed?

---

[16]https://www.fgdp.org.uk/sites/fgdp.org.uk/files/docs/in-practice/Research/critical_appraisal_pack.pdf

Impact factor of the journal

The impact factor is a measure of how frequently articles in the journal are cited. A higher impact factor suggests that the journal is more learned and has higher-quality content. One needs to remember, however, that it is also related to the specialty. Most specialist journals are likely to have lower impact factors than general medical journals, and subspecialty journals will have lower impact factors again.

Authors

- Which institution are they from? Is it a noteworthy academic institution?
- How many authors are there, e.g. is it a multicentre study with a lot of academic influence?
- Who are the authors? Are they renowned or credible in their field? Are there any non-academic or renowned statisticians in the list?
- Are the authors associated with drug/tech companies?
- Has the research been sponsored by an institution with a vested interest?

Submission

- How much time elapsed between original submission date and publication? In some papers the date of original submission is shown. A very long time between original submission and acceptance would suggest a lot of reworking.

Introduction

- Do the authors clearly lay out the background to the study as being worthy of investigation?
- Is the study particularly novel in comparison with what has already been published in the literature?
- Are the aims and hypothesis clearly set out?

Methods

Researchers may say this is the most important part of the paper, since this is the basis of the scientific approach that was used. This will vary depending on whether it is a case-controlled or cohort study (following up people over a period of time).

- What is the overall study design – case study, case-controlled, cohort study? Is this an interventional study, where a treatment or procedure is applied to one or more groups and results are measured subsequently?

  - If a review, was it systematic or a meta-analysis?
  - For a drug treatment or intervention, was it a randomised controlled trial?
  - For study of prognosis, was this a cohort study?
  - For study of causation, was this a case-controlled study?

- Was data collected prospectively or retrospectively? If retrospectively, it has greater chance for error if one is relying on data recorded prior to the conception of the study.

Although expert opinions exist in the literature, the main studies to be appraised would be those involving numerous subjects, i.e. case-controlled or cohort. In addition, the best form of evidence comes from meta-analyses, where randomised controlled trials (cohort) are compared. However, this involves complex statistics or calculations, to ensure that studies of often similar designs are presented in a comparable fashion. If you are required to comment on these, it would be more in terms of the suitability of the individual studies to be compared as a group and for you to interpret the final analysis, e.g. the combined odds or hazard ratios of an intervention, or risk on final outcome.

Case-controlled studies
- Was this a single-centred or multicentre study?
- Were there few or multiple study investigators?
- Were the case definitions and outcome measures accurately and appropriately defined?
- Were the clinical measures appropriately reproducible by all study measurements?
- Were cases appropriately matched to the controls? You may wish to look at subject characteristics such as demographics and other biometric values – are they explicitly documented in the report?

Randomised controlled trials (RCTs)
These are likely to form the majority of articles that you would be asked to appraise. Usually, they involve two or more study groups, followed up over time and differing only in the intervention (procedure or drug therapy they receive).

It is important that the study is well controlled and the groups differ only in the intervention. So:
- How were the subjects recruited? Was this random or consecutive?
- Are there any possibilities of bias in the recruitment process? Were measures added to specifically remove human choice and bias?
- What were the inclusion criteria? Did they include individuals who would innately bias the results of the intervention?
- What were the exclusion criteria? Did they exclude individuals for whom you would wish to know the impact of this intervention?
- Are the study groups large enough? The strength of any association will be measured statistically and this will depend on the size of the studies sampled. Often a "power" calculation is made before the study is undertaken, which guides the researchers in determining the optimum size of the study groups needed to reach a desired strength of significance.

- Was each of the study groups treated in the same way, with the exception of the intervention? This may include follow-up visits, number of measurements/investigations/scans, centre in which they receive their care, personnel they were in contact with, etc.
- Are the groups well matched for baseline characteristics? Often a table is shown detailing demographics and other biometric values – are there any characteristics missing from this table that you feel relevant, e.g. smoking or BMI?
- Was length of follow-up adequate? Some outcome measures are rare, and a long follow-up is required to await their manifestation.
- What were the study's end points (outcome measures) – were they appropriate for the question being asked? For example, periodontal disease measured by pocket depths, gingival bleeding, etc – was this the same for both groups? This may not be the case in a multicentre study.
- What was the dropout rate? Was this unacceptably high, thereby reducing the statistical power of those remaining in the study groups?
- How are dropouts and missing values accounted for statistically, i.e. was this an "on-treatment analysis", where only the results of those still on treatment at the end are evaluated; or is this an "intention to treat" analysis, where every subject's results are noted, whether they continued with the intervention or not? In this case the researchers have to decide what they do with subjects who changed intervention (switched drugs or interventions) or dropped out. This has to be clearly stated. A common example is "missed drug or intervention = failure". So, the number of dropouts will be relevant when studying the overall supposed effect in that study arm.

Results

- Are the results for all of the end points stated clearly (tabulated or graphically represented)?
- What statistical methods were used? Were they appropriate for the type of data collected, i.e. for continuous or discrete data – parametric or non-parametric methods?
- For data points in text, tables or graphs, were adequate confidence intervals calculated, i.e. to the 95% level? How wide are these confidence intervals? Is there overlap with the comparator groups?
- What is the *p*-value? This is the chance (between 0 and 1) that the observed event occurred by chance. By convention, a *p*-value less than 0.05 (i.e. a 1-in-20 chance) is deemed significant. Due reference should be paid to the sample size, as in smaller samples even a *p* value of <0.05 is irrelevant.
- Remember as well that statistically significant results are not necessarily *clinically* significant. The orthodontic bracket that tilts an incisor by an additional fraction of a degree is of no consequence for the patient on the receiving end!

Conclusions

The conclusion section should discuss only the findings stated in the results section. The authors must not present any new data in the conclusion section.

- The conclusions should be discussed in terms of association of the intervention or risk factor with the outcome measure. This association is only confirmed if the odds ratios of p-values are significantly strong, i.e. the usual cut-off for a p-value is less than 0.05, with the smallest p-values giving the greatest strength of association. Authors sometimes discuss "trends", where there is an apparent association in the data, yet the p-value is close to but not smaller than 0.05. It is acceptable for authors to state this, but one should be wary if most of their conclusions hang on trends of relatively large p-values.
- Some reviewers negatively critique papers in which many factors are analysed for association. These may be colloquially termed "fishing exercises", the criticism being (i) some of the positive findings were not the primary objectives of the study, and (ii) the more variables that are analysed from a data set, the greater the likelihood that an association may be found purely by chance. Be wary of post hoc analyses that trawl back through the data to find something publishable and present this as a significant finding, no matter what the statistics say!
- Where associations are strong, the authors will suggest a possible causation between intervention or risk factor and outcome measure. Are these causations scientifically plausible? Are they justified by putative mechanism of action or appropriate time relationship between cause and effect? Does this agree with findings of other research in this field?
- Do the authors make claims that you feel are appropriate or inappropriate regarding the evidence they have presented?
- Do they translate these findings to be applied to situations/populations, which you feel are reasonable or unreasonable?
- Are study limitations discussed? Are suggestions for future study refinement or extension work mentioned?
- Have appropriate plans been made for future study?

And finally

- Have the authors accepted or rejected their hypothesis, i.e. has this paper proven something to you? And crucially:
  - Does any of this apply to the populations or individuals you care for?
  - Will this change your management in any way?

9.29 Systematic review, meta-analysis and randomised controlled trials (RCTs)

Whilst discussing a paper, you may be asked probing questions about the different possible designs for research studies, such as "What is a randomised controlled trial?" or "What is a meta-analysis?" In this chapter we set out the different types of designs and their key features.

Systematic review and meta-analysis (evidence level Ia)

A systematic review is a review and summary of the existing high-quality research evidence relating to a given topic. Systematic reviews constitute the highest level of evidence for evidence-based dentistry purposes. There is a standardised method for conducting systematic reviews. Researchers will seek to include all relevant material, including non-English work, unpublished papers, and research from different databases. They will contact lead researchers and ask if they know of other publications that should be included.

Relevant studies are often combined, using meta-analysis. The best-known collection of systematic reviews is the Cochrane Collaboration.

A meta-analysis is a way of combining the results from several related studies into some form of standardised measure of effect size. By combining and adjusting the results from a collection of studies, giving appropriate weighting to the various studies involved, a meta-analysis will produce stronger evidence. On the negative side, the end result will only be as good as the material used for the meta-analysis – good meta-analysis of flawed research studies would result in flawed results.

Randomised controlled trial (evidence level Ib)

Randomised controlled trials (RCTs) are studies in which the interventions are randomly allocated to patients, in order to ensure that known and unknown confounding factors are evenly distributed between treatment groups. The word "controlled" refers to the fact that patients are not studied in isolation, but by reference to a "control group". The control group is given the old (or standard) treatment, a placebo that looks similar to the new treatment or no treatment at all.

Different types of control groups

- **No-treatment concurrent control groups** – subjects are randomly allocated the test treatment or no treatment.

- **Placebo concurrent control group** – Subjects are randomly allocated the test treatment, or a similar-looking treatment that does not contain the active element.

- **Active control group** – Subjects are randomly allocated the test treatment or another form of treatment. This type of control group tends to be used to demonstrate the superiority of one treatment over another.

- **Dose response control group** – Subjects are randomly allocated two different doses of the test treatment (this may include a zero dose, i.e. a placebo).

- **External control and historical control** – The test group is being compared with a group of patients who are external to the study. This may be a group of patients from an earlier study, or a group of patients treated contemporaneously but in a different setting.

- **Crossover trials** – The two treatments are switched between the two groups (after a washout period) to see which one has a better effect on any particular patient, i.e. the patient is the control.

Open vs. blind trials

- **Open trials** are trials where both the researcher and the patient knows which treatment the patient has been allocated. It is difficult to remove bias, since the patient knows whether or not he is being given a placebo. There are, however, situations where the patient needs to know what treatment is being administered, as does the clinician (for example, in the case of surgical procedures).

- **Single-blind trials** are trials where the researcher knows which treatment is being given to which patient, but where the patient does not know. The main drawback of this approach is that the researcher may subconsciously affect the outcome for the patient, treating and informing patients slightly differently in view of his/her knowledge.

- **Double-blind trials** are trials where neither the researcher nor the patient knows which treatment the patient has been allocated. Whenever there are viable alternatives, double-blind trials are the preferred option because they remove any bias. When the person administering the treatment is also unaware of which group the patient is in, this may be termed "triple-blind".

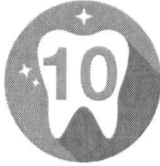

10 Difficult colleagues

What are the interviewers testing?

The interviewers will use these questions to test a range of skills and behaviours, including:

- Being safe: patients should be your first priority and the interviewers will want to know that you are not placing yourself or your colleagues before patient safety.

- Your understanding of the dilemmas that the situation presents: these questions are difficult because there isn't always a single answer. For example, there are rumours about a colleague taking drugs in his/her spare time. You could argue that it is none of your business, but it may develop into something more serious and place patients at risk. You will need to demonstrate that you understand the different perspectives and that you are able to decide on an appropriate course of action.

- Your approach to the problem: many candidates think that telling the clinical director will resolve the problem. There are often times, however, when the problem can be resolved without going to senior colleagues (e.g. if the subject has only been late a couple of times). In any case, seniors will generally prefer you to "bring solutions, rather than problems". There are times where it is necessary to involve a senior colleague, and this should be handled sensitively. The interviewers will be looking at the thought processes that you demonstrate.

- Your communication skills and empathy: some scenarios may contain a more human element, i.e. where the behaviour exhibited by the colleague is potentially linked to a personal problem. In other scenarios, the situation could be very delicate and seriously backfire if communication is not handled properly. The interviewers will be keen to know that you can handle these matters sensibly and communicate appropriately.

- Your team approach: it is unlikely that you will be able to sort out the problem by yourself. The interviewers will therefore want to determine to what extent you involve other people from the team, and how appropriate that involvement is.

Answering the question

Questions on problem colleagues may look different on the surface, but once you have learnt to answer a few of them, you will know how to approach pretty much any scenario thrown at you. In order to make best use of the material contained in this chapter, it is important that you familiarise yourself with the SPIES structure (see 5.3). It will form the backbone of your answer. In order to provide an effective answer, you will also need to follow the following principles:

Avoid providing answers that are too robotic and algorithmic
Although ready-made structures are extremely useful, to ensure that you don't forget any salient points, it is also crucial that you use your common sense whenever you answer any question relating to practical situations. You do not handle a drunken consultant in the same way that you would handle a junior colleague who is often late. Keep things in perspective and use your common sense.

Explain the "how" and the "why", not just the "what"
Most candidates "know" the answers to all these "difficult colleague" questions. However, not many deliver answers that are interesting to listen to. After 15 candidates, the interviewers will be bored of hearing the same thing, time after time. In order to provide an answer that is different and highlights your maturity, you will need to mention all the essential steps and why you would act that way.

For example, you may feel that the situation needs to be escalated to the clinical director. Why is that and how would you handle that process?

- Will you discuss the matter with the problem clinician first or not? If not, why not? And if yes, what will you be achieving by doing this?

- Is the clinical director the best person to contact? What about the colleague's educational supervisor or another consultant? Which is better and why?

- Will you actually be formally discussing the matter with a senior colleague, or will you simply raise it informally with them? Why? What are you seeking to achieve?

- You will no doubt need to demonstrate that you can support the colleague in question as well as your team in dealing with the problem. How will you do that and why?

My experience is that candidates take an approach that is far too theoretical when they answer questions on difficult colleagues. To ensure that your answer is natural, try to imagine what you would do if this were a real situation. In other words, stop thinking of the question as an "interview" question, and start picturing yourself in a real-life scenario. Use your common sense.

If possible, highlight the dilemmas at the start of your answer

Once you have been given a scenario, you should be able to determine very quickly what problems the situation poses. If possible, you should present these at the very start of the answer, so that your interviewers know how you are approaching the problem.

For example, if you have to deal with the "drunk consultant" question, you could start your answer with a statement such as "There are two problems that this scenario poses. I will need to make sure that patients are safe but I also need to make sure that the problem is handled sensitively so that the consultant does not suffer any more embarrassment than he has already caused."

This will give an idea of the direction that you are taking and will also reassure the interviewers that you are thinking rationally about the problem rather than just regurgitating some standard answer.

Avoid providing specific examples in the main body of the answer

Some of you may have had experience of dealing with problems similar to the scenario that the question is addressing. If this is the case, do not mention them before you have dealt with the generality of the question. If you go straight into a specific example, you will spend all your time on it and will miss out some vital parts of the answer, which may not have featured prominently in the real-life situation that you dealt with.

10.1 One of your consultants comes on the clinic drunk one morning. What do you do?

What you are trying to achieve?

Your main objectives in dealing with this situation will be to ensure that:

- Patient safety is assured.
- The consultant is safe.
- Seniors are aware so that action can be taken to prevent the problem from recurring, and to ensure that the issues which led the consultant to become drunk are being addressed.
- The consultant is supported in dealing with these issues.
- The whole situation is handled sensitively.

Applying the SPIES structure (see 5.3)

Seek information
There is little information you need to gather if you are actually present when the consultant comes in. The question is telling you that he/she is drunk, so there is no information you can gather that would make a difference to the way in which you handle the matter. The outcome of the investigation may, however, be altered if, for example, he/she has been affected temporarily by a divorce or bereavement.

Patient safety.
If the consultant is drunk, then he/she is a danger to patients and should be taken away from the clinical environment. The setting may be an outpatients consultation clinic in a dental hospital, a treatment session, a theatre list or a ward in a maxillofacial DCT interview ... the premise is the same with minor variations – patient safety takes priority!

There are many ways in which you could remove the consultant from the clinical area but, however you do it, you must make sure that you do it in the quickest and most sensitive manner, so as to minimise the impact on patients and the embarrassment to the consultant and to the team. Part of patient safety is the faith they have in the team and the profession as a whole.

You may want to try the following approaches (in decreasing order of suitability):
- Talk to the consultant and convince him/her to leave and go home.
- Involve another senior member of the team (another consultant or even a senior nurse) who may have more influence than you on the consultant. Remember

that you are trying to handle the matter sensitively, therefore you would need to involve someone that the consultant trusts in order to minimise conflict.
- Call on a senior member of an adjacent team. Typically, this would be another consultant.
- Summon the security team (as a very last resort – hopefully you will have found someone to help you before you reach this stage).

Once the consultant has left the clinical area, you will need to make sure that any actions or decisions made by that consultant are reviewed and that any patients he/she has seen are followed up appropriately.

Initiative

Is there any action that you could undertake by yourself (i.e. before you involve anyone else) to resolve or help the situation at your level? In the case of a drunken consultant, it would be inappropriate for you to attempt to resolve the entire problem by yourself; however, there are a number of useful steps that you can take such as:

- Make sure that the consultant is safe, i.e. that he/she goes home safely by taxi. Make sure that he/she doesn't drive home and check that he/she has arrived safely.

- Inform the person in charge that the consultant was unwell and needed to go home, so that appropriate cover can be arranged.

- Volunteer to cover some of consultant's duties, which might otherwise be neglected. At a junior level, you might not be able to take on the responsibilities that the consultant would have handled, but you can work with the team to share the workload and ensure that patient care is being appropriately provided.

Escalate

If the consultant turns up drunk, then there is no doubt that this shows a lack of insight – despite being drunk, he/she failed to realise that he/she could constitute a danger to patients. His/her judgement is questionable, and he/she therefore poses a risk to patients, not only in the present, but also in future if he/she has or develops an alcohol addiction.

As a result, you would be expected to raise the matter with an appropriate senior colleague. You would want to avoid contacting too many people so as not to spread rumours and undermine the reputation of the problem consultant. You really need to contact someone who is likely to have some influence over the situation; this would typically be the clinical director or a senior consultant, who can take the problem on board and start dealing with it.

From then on, you have effectively transferred the responsibility of dealing with the problem to senior colleagues. However, although this probably means that your input will no longer be required to deal with the core of the matter, you still have a responsibility to raise the alarm if you feel that the senior response is inadequate.

Support
The consultant's behaviour is likely to have its roots in some kind of personal problem. In addition, the incident is likely to have consequences, if not for his/her career, at least on his/her credibility. You should therefore show as much support as you can towards him/her (more so if you know him/her well). You should also ensure that you support your team in dealing with consequences of the problem; for example, you may need to take on extra duties temporarily until the consultant gets better (within limits of what would be commensurate with your level of training and with appropriate senior support and cover).

Follow-up questions

Interviewers often ask follow-up questions to test your understanding of your responsibilities and duties as a dentist. Follow-up questions typically include:

- "Once you have reported the problem to the clinical director, what is likely to happen?" (see 10.2)
- "What would you do if the drunken consultant asks you not to mention anything to anyone, because it was the first time that it happened and he/she promises it won't happen again?" (see 10.3)
- "If, after reporting the matter to the clinical director, you find that he/she is not responding appropriately, what would you do?" (see 10.4).

10.2 Once you have reported the problem to the clinical director, what is likely to happen?

This is a question which can be asked in many ways, either generally (i.e. according to the wording above) or more specifically (such as "Which external bodies is the clinical director likely to involve in order to resolve the situation?").

You can also structure the answer to this question according to the SPIES structure:

Seek information
The clinical director will want to gather information about the incident from you, from other colleagues who may have been present at the time and also from the consultant who was drunk. He/she will also want to learn, from others, whether similar incidents have occurred in the past.

Patient safety
The clinical director will need to make a decision as to the extent to which patient safety is endangered by the consultant and will need to take appropriate steps. This may include removing the consultant from certain duties or suspending him/her during the investigation. This is a decision that will need to be taken at trust level, following discussion with the medical director.

Initiative
The clinical director will need to ensure that patient care is covered adequately whilst the problem is being resolved. He/she will need to discuss with other colleagues how the team should be reorganised to deal with the consultant's enforced absence.

The clinical director will also seek to understand the reasons behind the consultant's behaviour. In particular, he/she should establish whether the problem is linked to some form of personal problem, stress at work or any other problem for which the consultant can be supported.

Escalate
In view of the seriousness of the incident, its potential impact on patient safety and on the reputation of the trust, the clinical director will most likely engage in a discussion with the medical director (i.e. his/her direct superior, who represents the clinical side on the trust's board). They will together, perhaps in consultation with the chief executive, decide how they should proceed. They may decide that the incident can be closed with a simple (but final) warning or they may move for suspension and reporting to the GDC.

Support

The level of support provided by seniors to the consultant will de
of the problem:

- Senior colleagues may be more understanding if there is a rea

- If the drinking has a personal cause (e.g. personal problems, stress at work), the clinical director may wish to offer support to the colleague to help him/her cope. This may include simply giving him/her additional time off, or even restructuring the way he/she works.

- If the drinking is a habit, then the clinical director should encourage the colleague to seek help from appropriate support groups. In some cases, this may even be a condition of the consultant's return to work.

10.3 What would you do if the drunken consultant asks you not to mention anything to anyone because it was the first time that it happened and he/she promises he/she won't happen again?

Your duty

The fact that he/she has turned up drunk raises concern about patient safety. Even if the consultant has not touched a single patient that day, the fact that he/she lacked insight about his/her own fitness to practise is worrying by itself. He/she should have recognised that he/she was unfit, called in sick and stayed at home. You therefore have no choice. You <u>must</u> report the matter to a senior colleague. Remember, patient safety here is your priority and you have a duty under GDC *Standards* Principles 8 – "Raise concerns if patients are at risk" – and 9 – "Make sure your personal behaviour maintains patients' confidence in you and the dental profession".

Communicating with the consultant

You are facing someone who is obviously trying hard to limit the damage that he/she has caused to him-/herself and you must be empathetic towards his/her situation. Whilst you should be firm in asserting that you have no choice, you should also try to be supportive and convey the message that, ultimately, if he/she has some form of problem, it will be best resolved with everything in the open. The best you can offer is your support and understanding.

Think of the worst-case scenario

Some candidates argue that "it is harsh to report someone if it is the first time they have made a mistake". If you think this, consider what would happen if the consultant came in drunk again, but this time harmed a patient. An investigation would be launched, and it would quickly be established that it had happened before, but that you kept quiet. This would get you into serious trouble and would do irreparable damage to the trust of patients in the department and profession as a whole, contravening the GDC principles outlined above. Therefore, you cannot take the risk, and you should report it to a senior colleague.

10.4 If, after reporting the matter to the clinical director, you find that he/she is not responding appropriately, what would you do?

A simple answer

If the clinical director/clinical lead is failing to act, then he/she may be unfit to practise because he/she is letting other clinicians potentially harm patients. Therefore, in accordance with the GDC's *Standards for the Dental Team*, you will need to report the matter to an appropriate senior colleague – in this case, the medical director for the trust. If the medical director fails, you will need to go to the chief executive, and after that to the GDC. This is the answer that most interviewers would be looking for and which, in most circumstances, would give you the maximum mark for this question.

However, although this would be an absolutely correct answer to give, some candidates have received feedback that the interviewers were looking for a "more refreshing answer". To provide a more comprehensive answer, you can use the SPIES structure.

A more comprehensive answer

Seek information
Accusations must be based on objective information. For example, you may have observed further patterns of unsafe behaviour. Make a note and enquire (discreetly) with other colleagues, if need be.

Patient safety
If there are further unsafe episodes, then you must ensure that patient safety is preserved. This may involve confronting the consultant about the recurrent problem. You may also have to discuss the problem with other senior colleagues.

Initiative
The fact that you believe that the clinical director is not responding appropriately does not actually mean that he/she has been completely ignoring the problem. He/she may have tried to resolve the problem, but struggled to deal with that consultant and be currently working on alternative plans. You should not jump to conclusions. If you remain concerned about the perceived lack of progress, it would be appropriate to return to the clinical director and ask what has happened. The clinical director might then explain to you how he/she is handling the situation. If you feel that your concerns are not being taken seriously, then you should escalate.

Escalate

If you feel that you are being ignored or that the action taken is insufficient, then you need to take your concerns to the medical director and, if necessary, to the chief executive.

Whatever you do, never escalate without having first exhausted discussions at each level. For example, if you have a problem with the clinical director, raise it with him/her first before going to the medical director. Also, never raise your concerns with people like the media, as you would undermine the authority of your superiors (those who genuinely care) and you may also undermine patient confidence in their local/regional dental hospital / clinic / acute hospital. This would be counterproductive, and you may in fact make things worse overall.

If you do not know how to handle the issue, then you can seek advice from your defence union, Practitioner Performance Advice (formerly NCAS), British Dental Association or even the GDC.

Support

Ultimately, patient care is what matters most; so you should continue to support your team in dealing with patients, despite all the problems that are taking place. You should also continue to support the problem clinician.

10.5 One of your junior colleagues has been late for 20 minutes every day for the past four days. What do you do?

This is another question about a problem colleague, and therefore we suggest using the SPIES structure.

Seek information
There may be different reasons why the colleague is late. Maybe he/she has discussed this with a senior colleague previously but simply failed to inform you about it. Maybe he/she is having personal problems, which he/she does not wish to share with others. Maybe his/her train is late due to engineering works. Maybe he/she is new to the hospital and is travelling long distances. Or maybe he/she has an attitude problem.

With a lot of "maybes", you really need to seek some information about the nature of the problem. This can be done by approaching the colleague and gently asking whether there is anything you can help with. You can add that you have noticed he/she has had trouble getting to work on time.

Patient safety
A delay of 20 minutes is unlikely to cause major concern towards patient safety. In most cases, it will have an impact on the team without necessarily impacting on safety. However, there may be cause for concern if:

- The colleague is missing handovers and provides substandard care.
- The colleague rushes jobs to make up for his/her lateness.
- There are issues with continuity of care due to patients being picked up by colleagues, e.g. orthodontic review appointments for appliance adjustments.

If this is the case, then you should raise these concerns with a clinic or ward manager or any senior colleague, so that they can take action. You should also ensure that patient safety is not affected. This may mean ensuring that you take on some of his/her jobs or place at handovers.

Initiative
It is possible that the problem is due to a temporary problem such as family problems or train delays. If the problem is likely to be very short-term and you are reassured that your colleague has tried his/her best to sort things out, then you may wish to show a little flexibility by covering for him/her for the period of the delay and also by recommending that he/she should discuss his/her problems with a senior colleague or a manager, so that they can arrange a more flexible working pattern

temporarily. Whatever you agree with your colleague should be shared with someone more senior. The manager may suggest a contract that makes expectations transparent for both parties.

Escalate

If you feel that the problem is affecting patient safety, that there is a lack of insight or that it is likely to persist, you will need to involve a consultant more formally.

Support

If the issue is linked to a family problem, then your colleague will appreciate your personal support during this difficult period.

The answer to this question requires more consideration than for the underperforming colleague. Due to the strong likelihood that the delay is linked to personal issues, your answer should reflect this by placing an equal emphasis on flexibility and support, and on raising the matter with senior colleagues.

10.6 Whilst in the office, you see a bag of what looks like cocaine drop from your registrar's pocket. What do you do?

This question works along a similar line to the others (i.e. you can answer it using the SPIES structure (see 5.3) except that, this time, you only have a suspicion rather than actual proof).

Dealing with the lack of certainty

When you deal with a drunken colleague, the impact on patient safety is clear and, once you have ensured that patients are safe, you need to report your concerns. However, in the case of a bag of cocaine falling out of your registrar's pocket, there are some unknowns; for example:

- Is it actually cocaine? You could of course enquire with your colleague but he/she is unlikely to own up to it.
- Assuming it is cocaine, is your colleague actually taking any? He/she could be carrying it for someone else. He/she might even be selling it on.

You don't know whether this matter is impacting on patient care and your colleague's safety as a dentist. For this reason, you cannot take the risk of letting the matter go and, on the basis that you are not the best person to investigate this issue, you will need to report it to senior colleagues. If, after investigation, the matter is nothing to worry about (maybe it was just sweetener!), then everyone will just move on. However, if the matter is serious, then the seniors will be able to handle it properly because you have brought it to their attention.

"Raising the matter with seniors seems harsh"

Some may argue that reporting the matter with seniors is harsh. It may be the case (particularly if it was not cocaine, after all), but you need to weigh this against the alternatives. Sorting this out directly with the colleague will most likely lead you nowhere (since he/she will undoubtedly deny it) and, in any case, it would only lead to a temporary solution (you can't keep an eye on the colleague every single day – it is not your job). Doing nothing would actually be unsafe. Not only might he/she be under the effects of cocaine at work, but also the drug abuse may be linked to stress or personal problems. These may be affecting your colleague's performance. Your success in handling the matter well will rest in the sensitivity that you demonstrate through your communication with everyone involved.

10.7 You wrote a case report for publication, which you gave to a consultant for review. After two weeks, he/she gives it back to you with two additional author names: his/her brother's and his/her spouse's. What do you do?

Issues raised by the question

The issues in this question are as follows:

- The consultant lacks integrity by adding the names of two people (his/her brother and spouse), who not only have not contributed to the case (if they did contribute to the case then there is absolutely no problem), but also are two other clinicians out there who have CVs with potentially fake information and may be getting jobs under false pretences. The fact that it is only a case report may not seem a big deal, but this indicates a certain frame of mind and they may well be faking other aspects of their CVs. This does not reflect well on the consultant's integrity as a healthcare professional.

- Having more authors undermines your own efforts as it dilutes your involvement.

On both counts, patient safety is not immediately affected, i.e. there is no reason to act that very minute, but it does raise some important questions. The best way to deal with it is as follows (following the SPIES structure):

Seek information
Discuss with the consultant why he/she has added the two names. Raise your concerns and try to get a sensible explanation from him/her.

Patient safety
No immediate action required. Patient safety is not immediately affected.

Initiative
Try to convince the consultant that this is wrong. Try to get him/her to change his/her mind. If you can, you should stand your ground and insist that the names are taken off. If the consultant has already given you the corrections back, then you may take the initiative to send the case report off to the journal without the two names in question.

Escalate

If the situation is not easily resolved, then you may consider raising the issue with another consultant or the clinical director.

Support

Not relevant here.

Follow-up question

Whenever candidates have been asked this question, it was followed up by the following question: "The consultant is your referee and may give you a bad reference if you contest. How do you handle the situation?"

In answer to this question, if you are really worried about your reference, then you need to discuss the matter with someone else at a senior level. They should arrange for another referee to take over. If there is no time to arrange another referee, they should discuss the reference with the consultant in question beforehand, to make sure that you do not suffer from the consequences.

10.8 Your consultant is managing a patient against the recommendations of the established guidelines. What do you do?

This question looks like a question on a difficult consultant but combines it with your knowledge of evidence-based practice and, more specifically, your understanding of the definition of a "guideline" (see 9.27).

Seek information

Before you jump to conclusions, you need to understand why the consultant is making the decision to go against the guideline. After all, he/she has several more years' experience and his/her decision is most likely to be correct.

The process of evidence-based dentistry combines many more aspects than just the guideline. In particular, the consultant's clinical judgement and the patient's values have to be taken into account. Consequently, there are many reasons why the consultant may have taken his/her decision. For example:

- The guideline may not be suitable for the patient.
- The consultant may be aware of recent evidence that would supersede the guideline (though the guideline has not yet been changed to allow for that evidence).
- The guideline may be suitable, but the patient may have refused the recommended treatment.

Whatever the situation, the consultant should be in a position to educate you about his/her decision. The easiest way to approach him/her without sounding confrontational is to raise with him/her the fact that you are struggling to understand the decision that is being made and would like to discuss it with the consultant from an educational perspective.

Hopefully, by that time, you will be reassured that he/she is making the right decision.

Ensure patient safety at all costs; escalate if necessary

If, after obtaining further information from the consultant, you feel uncomfortable about the proposed management, then you must raise your concerns: in the first instance with the consultant, and, if needed, with another consultant. If you cannot get hold of another consultant, talk to the clinical director or another colleague.

Don't forget that you could also be wrong. So, if you have doubts, you always have the opportunity to discuss the issue with colleagues at your level or look things up.

Also, remember not to contradict the consultant in front of patients. Any disagreement should be raised away from patients.

If the situation is an emergency and you do not have time to ask for a second opinion or engage in a discussion, then you will have no choice but to let the consultant go with his/her decision, but you <u>must</u> record your disagreement in writing in the patient notes. This way, if there is a problem, you will not be blamed for not trying to resolve the initial problem. You should do this from an independent perspective, however, and not in written correspondence with third parties for the time being.

Learn from the situation
If the consultant ended up being correct, then you must ensure that you take steps to learn from that situation. You might want to read up on related matters or discuss the case at a teaching session.

10.9 Your consultant has made a mistake as a result of an error of judgement and is asking you to alter the patient's notes to match his/her version of events. What do you do?

There is no possible motive that could justify the consultant's behaviour. By not reporting the matter, you would not only help the consultant cover up for his/her mistake but you would also expose other patients to harm by not ensuring that action is taken against the consultant.

Seek information
There is no information to gather here, as the nature of the problem is obvious.

Patient safety
Ensure that whatever mistake has been committed has been resolved and that the patient is safe (if the mistake did not result in death).

Initiative
Refuse to comply with the consultant's request and explain that it is unethical. You should also make a written record of the conversation that you are having with the consultant, as your testimony may be required if any further action is taken.

Escalate
This issue is too serious for you to handle on your own. The consultant's behaviour is placing patients at risk and poses questions about his/her integrity. You should report the matter to the clinical director at the first opportunity. If he/she is not available or refuses to deal with the issue, escalate the matter to the medical director and thereafter to the chief executive.

Support
There is no support to give here, other than maybe towards the team in dealing with a situation where a consultant has gone (since he/he will most likely be suspended if your claims prove true).

10.10 During a clinic, your consultant shouts at you in front of a patient for getting an answer wrong. What do you do?

This is the type of question where it can be easy to get into automatic mode without thinking about the depth of the question, with an answer such as "This is bullying and therefore I will need to report it".

Yes, technically it is bullying, and yes, it is unacceptable. However, your reaction will much depend on who the consultant is, whether he/she makes a habit of it, or whether it was just a normally pleasant consultant who became irritated on that day because of stress.

In your answer, you will therefore need to ensure that the unacceptability of the event is addressed, but also that you place the whole event into perspective and use your common sense.

Seek information
It is best not to allow the situation to escalate to full conflict, particularly in front of patients. In the first instance, you should simply shut up and arrange to meet the consultant after the clinic so that any discussion can be held in private. This will ensure that patients do not become witnesses to more conflict and also that an adult discussion can take place away from the emotions of the argument that took place in front of others. Once you are with the consultant, you must insist on an explanation for the shouting.

Patient safety
There is no patient "safety" issue as such here, but the patient's confidence in their dental care may have been undermined by the argument that they witnessed. You have also been embarrassed by the incident. In such circumstances, it would be appropriate for the consultant to talk to the patient themselves, to apologise and reassure them. If the consultant does not want to do this, then you should take the initiative to do so yourself. If you feel uncomfortable about the whole idea or you feel that you may make things worse, you always have the option to talk to another consultant about it, who may be able to assist in the process.

Initiative
During the discussion with the consultant, if he/she has identified areas of concern about your performance, you should ask him/her how he/she feels you can resolve this. However, you should also remind him/her that it is never acceptable to put someone down in public, and even less so in front of patients. If you feel that you cannot do this, perhaps because the consultant is aggressive generally anyway, and

that raising the matter directly with him/her would be counterproductive, then you still have the option of asking another consultant for advice (such as your educational supervisor, or any other consultant).

Escalate

If you feel threatened by the consultant or if this incident has become a bit of a habit, then you have to ensure that you discuss the problem with senior colleagues. In the first instance, the most obvious port of call would be your educational supervisor for advice, but you really ought to go straight to the clinical director as he/she is the person who is likely to have the most influence on the situation in terms of finding a lasting solution.

If this fails, then you should refer to the section in your employee manual/booklet dealing with bullying. That section will most likely tell you to report the matter in confidence, either to the medical director or to someone from HR (each trust is likely to have its own policy).

However, one thing is for sure: before you escalate the matter outside of your team, you must take all possible steps to demonstrate that you have attempted to resolve the problem amicably within your team.

Support

This is not so relevant here. If anything, you are the one who needs to be supported. However, if the shouting was linked to stress or personal problems on the consultant's side, then you should show some understanding (which is different from accepting the bullying!).

It is worth noting that there are many trainee-led initiatives happening in medicine and surgery to counteract bullying in the workplace (e.g. the "Hammer it Out" campaign by the British Orthopaedic Trainees Association (BOTA)), and that dentistry and dental training programmes are beginning to follow suit in the recognition and ability to deal with this problem.[17]

---

[17] O'Dowd A. Health service staff stress rising amid plans for mental wellbeing help. *Br Dent J* 2019;226:389

10.11 Your consultant does not seem interested in providing you with appropriate teaching. What do you do?

This question is perhaps more subtle than any other because it is nothing to do with clinical underperformance and immediate patient safety. Although the consultant is obviously not fulfilling his/her duties, the resolution of the problem will be a test of your communication skills and initiative more than your willingness to report the consultant quickly.

Seek information
There are a few reasons why the consultant may not be providing appropriate teaching. Either he/she just can't be bothered, or he/she is otherwise engaged and is finding it difficult to fit everything in. Maybe the consultant is in the early throes of his/her career and still "finding his/her feet" and therefore less able/confident to teach or delegate.

Your first step will therefore be to determine the reasons why he/she is not providing any teaching. This is best addressed directly with the consultant in question. Because this is a teaching matter, you may first want to get together with other trainees to discuss the problem so that one of you approaches him/her with a mandate on behalf of the others. It may prove counterproductive to approach the consultant as a group because he/she may feel that you are ganging up on him/her.

Patient safety
Patient safety is not directly affected by the lack of teaching (in fact, you probably spend more time with patients than you should), so there is no action needed on that front. It is worth giving a nod to the fact that the ultimate aim of a training programme is to produce an independent specialist and so thinking further down the track, patient safety could potentially become an issue if you pass your training "on paper" but with insufficient clinical exposure and responsibility.

Initiative
Once you have organised a discussion with the consultant, you need to explain what you perceive the problem to be. This could be a simple lack of teaching time, a lack of protected time, or the fact that the teaching is there but lacks depth. During the discussion, you must acknowledge the constraints placed upon the department in relation to teaching and avoid being over-critical. You must show a willingness to engage with the senior team to find a solution to the problem. Never forget that your aim is to find a solution to your problem, not to engage in confrontation for the sake of it.

In parallel to all this, you must show appropriate initiative to compensate for the lack of teaching, by organising teaching with other consultants if you can, and by getting together with other trainees to organise study groups (if you are studying for exams, for example). It is of course important to get the problem consultant to provide teaching, but you cannot afford to wait until the problem is resolved to start training, as you will waste your entire attachment.

So, until the situation improves, make sure that you organise your own solutions too. In doing so, you will need to involve other registrars or consultants anyway, which may provide a wake-up call to the team about the problem consultant.

Escalate

If, despite your best (and constructive) efforts, the situation is not evolving, then you should broaden the discussion by involving your educational supervisor and perhaps other consultants. One idea may be to raise the matter of teaching in general at a team meeting (e.g. clinical governance meeting), avoiding mentioning the consultant in question but trying to get all seniors to agree on a training structure that is compatible with the level of service that needs to be provided to patients.

If the matter is stalling, then you should also involve your clinical director, either directly or, preferably, through your educational supervisor (since he/she is responsible for your education and is also a consultant, which makes him/her an ideal person to deal with other consultants).

Support

There is no real support that needs to be brought to the consultant here, unless the lack of teaching is due to the fact that he/she is overstretched in other areas, in which case you may consider helping the team restructure its work so that the consultant's workload is alleviated.

In answering this question, the emphasis should be on discussion and negotiation. Make sure that you escalate to the appropriate people and do not escalate until you have tried every step to make the situation improve, with the consultant first, and then your educational supervisor.

10.12 You see one of your colleagues looking at child pornography on the clinic computer. What do you do?

This question can be dealt with successfully using the SPIES structure (see 5.3).

Seek information

Child pornography is not only illegal, but your colleague also represents a possible danger to patients. Because of the seriousness of the situation, the issue will most certainly need to be discussed with a senior colleague. However, before you go down that route, you ought to discuss with the colleague in question what you saw. It may be a misunderstanding (i.e. perhaps it was simply a spam email that he/she received and opened, or perhaps a pop-up that he/she could not control), but it is difficult for you to investigate.

Patient safety

There is an obvious paediatric patient safety issue here, though it may not be immediate if the colleague is often working supervised or with other healthcare professionals. To ensure patient safety, for the immediate future, you should reassure yourself that the dentist is never on his/her own. You should also ensure that the matter is reported to a senior colleague as soon as possible so that further measures can be taken appropriately (e.g. suspension).

Initiative

So far, you have taken as much initiative as you could. Many candidates know that, for this question, the police need to be involved (since it is criminal), but this will really be a matter for the trust to handle rather than you. By calling the police yourself, you may cause more harm than good in the short term (imagine the impact on your team and the patients if the police turned up on the ward to arrest the dentist in question!).

Escalate

Based on the above, your main responsibility will be to report the matter to a consultant or the clinical director as soon as possible. If the colleague is a consultant, then you should go to the clinical director. If the colleague is the clinical director, then you should talk to the medical director. The seniors will deal with the matter, including ensuring that the police are being called, but you will need to make sure that this is in hand and take appropriate measures if for any reason this does not follow through (see 10.4).

Support

You may provide personal support to him/her through this ordeal and you should ensure that the matter is handled sensitively and confidentially.

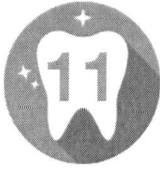

11 Confidentiality, consent and other ethical principles

Occasionally, you may be asked questions relating to general ethics and its application to concrete scenarios. These questions could relate to issues as varied as difficult patients, complex consent issues, or the management of an emergency with which you are unfamiliar.

The range of possible questions has no boundaries, and your knowledge of ethics can be tested in different ways:

- By asking you factual questions about a key issue:
    - "What do you understand by the words 'Gillick competence'?"
    - "In which circumstances do you think it is acceptable to breach patient confidentiality?"

- By asking you how you would handle a specific situation, e.g.:
    - A 14-year-old girl attending for emergency treatment for dental trauma without an accompanying adult
    - Signs of non-accidental injury (NAI) in a paediatric dentistry patient

- By engaging you in role play, with the patient being played by an interviewer or a trained actor

Whatever the format, it is helpful to remember that all issues relate to four key principles. Therefore, rather than learn the management of individual situations by heart, concentrate on understanding and applying those key principles.

11.1 The four ethical principles of biomedical ethics

The following four principles are those used in biomedical science to guide decisions:

Beneficence
This word comes from the Latin "Bene" = good, and "Facere" = to do. Essentially, it means that you must act in the patient's best interest.

Non-maleficence (also, but rarely, called "non-malfeasance")
From the Latin "Male" = bad, and "Facere" = to do. You must not harm your patients. It is important to remember that many treatments may actually harm the patient (e.g. through side effects), but what you need to keep in mind is the balance between benefit and harm.

Autonomy
From the Greek words "Auto" = self, and "Nomos" = law, custom.
The patient has the right to choose what they want (i.e. whether to accept or refuse treatment).

Justice
Patients must be treated fairly. This principle deals mainly with the distribution of scarce resources and is particularly relevant when dealing with expensive drugs or procedures. It is the principle that may be applied to justify not giving a patient an expensive treatment, if it means that a large number of patients then cannot benefit from other treatments as a result. Recent discussions surrounding the commissioning of orthognathic surgery and the place of the index of orthognathic functional treatment need (IOFTN) in stratifying treatment need come to mind here.

Whenever a dilemma occurs, it is because two or more of these principles clash. For example, a Jehovah's Witness refusing a blood transfusion will cause a clash between:

- Beneficence – transfusing is the best option to manage the patient
- Non-maleficence – not transfusing may result in the patient's death
- Autonomy – the patient can choose what they feel is best for them

Note: If the patient is competent, autonomy always prevails over beneficence and non-maleficence, i.e. the patient can do what they want with their body, whether you think it will benefit them or harm them.

11.2 Confidentiality

The patient's right to confidentiality

The right to confidentiality is central to the dentist–patient relationship and is enshrined in GDC *Standards* Principle 4 – Maintain and protect patients' information. It creates trust, which makes patients feel safe to share information, without fear of that information being used inappropriately.

There are simple measures that you can implement to ensure that patient confidentiality is protected (some of which may be discussed at interviews in specific patient-based scenarios). These include:

- Not leaving computers with patient records unattended
- Not leaving patient details showing on screen where they can be viewed by others
- Not letting patient notes lie around and not taking notes home with you unless they have been anonymised
- Not leaving handover sheets where they can be seen by patients and families
- Ensuring you check the identity of patients, particularly if you are discussing matters over the phone
- If the patient comes accompanied, asking the patient if they are comfortable with a third person sitting in on the consultation
- Not using the public as translators, even if they offer (e.g. unaccompanied, non-English speaker attending for emergency dental treatment). There are a number of commercial interpreters available via telephone (e.g. LanguageLine Solutions)
- Carefully considering your reactions to questions asked by relatives or outside organisations (police, social services, etc) when directed towards you

The Information Commissioner's Office (ICO) *Guide to the General Data Protection Regulation (GDPR)* is a good source of information here and is available online.[17]

Breaching patient confidentiality

Although patient confidentiality should be protected, there may be instances where it needs to be breached, some of which may be relevant to your daily practice.

The situations where breaching confidentiality is appropriate include:

---

[17]https://ico.org.uk/for-organisations/guide-to-data-protection/guide-to-the-general-data-protection-regulation-gdpr/

- **Sharing information with other healthcare professionals or others involved in the care of the patient**

  As a dentist, you constantly breach patient confidentiality by passing on information to other healthcare professionals. This may include sending a letter of correspondence to the patient's GP and/or GDP, or sending a referral letter to another clinician in secondary or tertiary care. It is accepted that such breaches are a routine aspect of patient management, providing the information is restricted to essential information. The patient is deemed to have provided implied consent. However, you must make sure that the patient understands that such disclosure of information is being made and, if the patient objects to the disclosure, you must take every possible step to comply with their wishes.

- **Using information for the purpose of clinical audit**

  For the results of clinical audits to be meaningful, they need to include a representative sample of the patient cohort. Providing that patients have been informed that their data may be used internally for the purpose of audit and healthcare improvement, and providing they have not objected to its use, then you may use their data for the purpose of audit. This is a form of implied consent, since you are not actually asking the patient to agree; you are simply informing them and allowing them to disagree, which rarely happens. If data is being given to external organisations for audit purposes, then the data must be anonymised. GDPR also governs the way data is stored. Patients need to be informed of which personal details are being held for audit or research purposes.

- **Disclosures required by law**

  There are a number of statutory requirements such as notifying a communicable disease, in accordance with the Public Health (Infectious Diseases) Regulations 1988. This includes measles, meningitis, mumps, tetanus and many others. The full list is available from the Health Protection Agency's website.[18] As always, you should make every effort to inform the patient, but their refusal cannot discharge you from your legal obligations.

- **Court order**

  You must disclose any information requested through a court order.

- **Disclosures to a statutory regulatory body**

  When investigating the fitness to practise of a health professional, regulatory bodies may require information about specific patient cases. Whenever possible, you should discuss the disclosure of the information with the patients concerned. If discussing consent is not practical, or the patient refuses to give consent, then you need to discuss the situation with the regulatory body in

---

[18] www.hpa.org.uk

question (e.g. GDC). They may judge that the disclosure is justified, even without patient consent.

- **Disclosure in the public interest and to protect the patient or others from risk of serious harm or death**
  There may be cases where the benefit to society far outweighs the harm to the patient caused by the release of information:

  - In extreme cases of HIV patients knowingly infecting others
  - An epileptic driver who continues to drive, despite advice from the DVLA
  - Any case of very serious abuse, where the victim is at serious risk of harm or death, even if they are a competent adult
  - Notifying the presence of a sex offender
  - A patient who is a healthcare professional placing patients at risk through a medical condition (e.g. a dental surgeon with hepatitis C)

- **Treatment of children or incompetent adults**
  This may happen when a child comes to see you, is not competent enough to make a decision, but is asking you to keep their visit confidential (the same would apply to any incompetent adult). In the first instance, you will need to negotiate with the patient, to convince them to involve an appropriate person. If they refuse, then you may need to involve a third party anyway, but only if you consider that the treatment is essential and in the patient's best interest. The patient should be aware of your intentions at all times.

- **Abuse or neglect of an incompetent person**
  The most common cases would be child or elderly abuse, or abuse of a patient with a mental illness. If disclosure is in the best interest of the patient, then you should do so promptly. If you decide not to report, you should be able to justify your decision. In fact, with child abuse, there is a duty to share information with other agencies, such as social care and the police. Therefore, if you suspect a child is about to make a disclosure, you should inform them that you will keep information confidential, unless they tell you something that you would need to share in order to protect their best interests.

Involving the patient

Whenever you need to breach confidentiality, you should always discuss it with the patient beforehand, obtain their consent and inform them of your plan. Although potentially a difficult conversation, it would certainly be easier than having to explain the breach afterwards. Being open and honest is generally appreciated by patients, even in challenging situations.

11.3 Competence and capacity

The difference between competence and capacity

Consent can only be taken from patients who are deemed to be "competent", i.e. who understand the information and are capable of making a rational decision by themselves. Competence is a legal judgement.

Healthcare professionals also frequently talk about "capacity to consent" or "mental capacity". This is a clinical judgement. Capacity is formally assessed by healthcare professionals, who must be sure that a patient is able to understand the proposed management, to comprehend the risks and benefits and to retain that information long enough to make balanced choices.

Because "competence" and "capacity" have similar meanings (in effect, a judge would rule as "competent" someone who has the capacity to make decisions concerning their care), most clinicians use them interchangeably.

Both competence and capacity are situation and time-specific, i.e. they are determined at a particular point in time, in relation to a given treatment or procedure. So, for example, a patient may be competent enough to decide whether they agree to have periodontal charting, but not whether they should go ahead with a full dental clearance under general anaesthesia.

Determining if someone has capacity to consent / is competent

Before you can obtain consent from a patient, you must ensure that they are competent, i.e. that they have the capacity to make the decision to go ahead with the proposed treatment or procedure.

The assessment of mental capacity should be made in accordance with the Mental Capacity Act 2005 (or the Adults with Incapacity Act 2000 in Scotland). Essentially, a patient is considered to have capacity if he/she:

• Understands the information provided in relation to the decision that needs to be made
• Is able to retain the information
• Is able to use and weigh up the information
• Can communicate his/her decision, by whatever means possible.

Every adult is presumed to have capacity

English law dictates that every adult should be assumed to have capacity to consent, unless proven otherwise. Essentially, this means that the patient retains full control of decisions affecting his/her care (i.e. his/her autonomy), unless someone challenges this assumption and conclusively proves otherwise.

A seemingly irrational decision does not imply lack of capacity

If a patient makes a decision that you consider irrational (such as refuses removal of carious, unrestorable teeth causing recurrent infections), it does not mean that they lack capacity. Similarly, you should not presume that someone is incompetent because they have a mental illness, are too young, can't communicate easily, have beliefs that go against yours or make decisions with which you disagree.

If you are unsure about your assessment

There may be situations where you are unsure as to whether a patient should be considered to have capacity to consent or not. In such cases, you should:

- Ask the opinion of colleagues, who may have a longer-term relationship with the patient concerned e.g. GP, GDP
- Involve colleagues with more specialist knowledge such as a psychiatrist or a neurologist

Some hospitals have a clinical ethics team, who can consider the particulars of the case and advise. If you are still unsure, you should seek legal advice, as a court may need to make that decision.

A good reference work for the place of the Mental Capacity Act 2005 in the provision of dental care is Emmett C. The Mental Capacity Act 2005 and its impact on dental practice. *Br Dent J* 2007;203:515–521. Many indemnity insurance providers also provide good overviews on their websites.

11.4 Seeking informed consent from a competent patient

Definition of informed consent

Informed consent is the agreement, granted by a patient, to receive a given treatment, or have a specified procedure performed on them, in full consideration of the facts and implications. The following sections summarise the key issues that you need to be aware of for your interview.

Basic model to obtain informed consent from competent patients

When the patient is competent, seeking informed consent is a relatively straightforward process, as follows:

Step 1: The patient and the dentist discuss the presenting complaint. During the consultation, the dentist gauges the level of understanding of the patient, takes account of their views and values, and presents a range of possible management options.

Step 2: The dentist describes the available options, including:
- Diagnosis and prognosis, including degree of certainty and further investigations required
- Different management options available to the patient, including the outcome of receiving no treatment. It is likely that the dentist will recommend a preferred course of action, but he should in no circumstances coerce the patient
- Details of any necessary investigations/treatments and/or procedures, including their purpose, their nature and which professionals will be involved
- Details of the risks, benefits, side effects and likelihood of success. The dentist should inform the patient of any serious possible risks (e.g. loss of the tooth/teeth, permanent altered/loss of sensation) even if the likelihood of occurrence is very small. He should also inform the patient about less serious side effects or complications if they occur frequently
- Whether the procedure or treatment is part of a research programme or innovative treatment, as well as the patient's right to refuse to participate in research or teaching projects
- Their right to a second opinion

- Any treatment that you or your organisation cannot provide, but which may be of greater benefit to the patient. This may include procedures for which no one has been trained in your organisation, or treatments not provided by your organisation on grounds of cost, but which may be provided elsewhere.

The information should be provided using terms that the patient can understand, and the dentist should check the understanding of the patient, answering the patient's questions as appropriate. When asked questions, the dentist should endeavour to respond in the most informative manner, avoiding coercion. If necessary, the dentist should use all necessary means of communication, including visual aids, leaflets, and models.

Step 3: The patient weighs up the benefits and risks and determines whether to accept or refuse the proposed options. If the patient refuses, then the dentist should explore their reasons and continue the discussion as long as the patient wants to. There may be concerns that were not identified or addressed previously. The dentist should inform the patient that they have the right to a second opinion and the opportunity to change their mind later on, if they so wish.

There are circumstances when modifications may be necessary during the primary planned procedure (e.g. bone grafting at the time of implant placement, apparent on direct inspection of the surgical site; pulpal exposure; and need for endodontic treatment in placing deep restorations). You need to explain these anticipated alterations to the patient clearly and obtain consent for these potential procedures.

Who should seek consent from the patient?

The responsibility to seek consent from the patient rests with the clinician who is proposing the treatment or will be carrying out the procedure. It is possible to delegate the task to someone else, but only if the person seeking the consent is suitably trained and qualified and they have appropriate knowledge of the treatment/procedure and the associated risks (e.g. trainee grades taking consent for a day case dentoalveolar general anaesthetic list). Although the task of consenting is delegated, the responsibility still rests with the clinician who is proposing the treatment or doing the procedure.

Verbal vs. written consent

The importance of recording consent is to demonstrate that the process took place with due care and diligence, and that both parties had a shared vision of the proposed procedure and any key complications.

In many cases, implied or verbal consent is sufficient. For example, if a patient opens their mouth so that you can examine them, their compliance constitutes consent.

For simple or routine procedures, investigations or treatment (e.g. examinations, bitewing radiographs), verbal consent may be sufficient. However, you must make sure that the patient has properly understood the information provided and has taken an informed decision. You should also ensure that their consent is duly recorded in their notes, together with the information on which it was based.

You should get written consent:

- For complex or more involved procedures
- If there are serious risks involved
- If there are potential consequences for the patient's employment, or social or personal life
- When providing clinical care is not the primary purpose of the investigation or procedure
- When the treatment is part of a research or innovative programme

11.5 Dealing with a patient who lacks capacity

When a patient lacks capacity, the dentist must provide care that is in the patient's best interest. It is preferable for the patient to be as involved as they can be in any discussion about their care. This consideration will be particularly pertinent for special care dentistry.

Whatever decisions are being taken by the dentist, the patient should be treated with respect and dignity, and should not be discriminated against. In making decisions on behalf of the patient, the dentist should take account of a wide range of issues, including:

• Whether the patient has signed an advance directive stating how he wants to be treated in situations when he can't give informed consent

• The views of any individuals who are legally representing the patient or whom the patient has said they wanted to involve

• The views of any individuals who are close to the patient (e.g. their relatives) and may be able to comment on their beliefs, values and feelings

• Whether the lack of capacity is temporary (e.g. the patient may be temporarily unconscious) or permanent

Unless the patient has signed an advance directive, the management decisions will rest with the dentist. Legally, relatives and others have only an advisory role. In practice, the dentist should try to seek a consensus around the care of the patient by involving all relevant parties in the discussions.

Sometimes there are disagreements, either between clinicians / healthcare professionals involved in the care of the patient as part of a multidisciplinary team, or between the dental team and those close to the patient. In situations such as these, it is important to seek conflict resolution through negotiation. Useful resources could include consulting more experienced colleagues, or using mediation services or independent advocates. In cases of more severe disagreements, then legal advice should be sought and a court decision may be needed.

11.6 Competence/capacity in children

Can children give informed consent?

All children aged 16 or above can be assumed to be competent, i.e. they can essentially be treated in exactly the same way as adults. Children under the age of 16 can give consent to a treatment, procedure or investigation if they are deemed to be Gillick competent, in reference to a famous House of Lords ruling on the ability of children under 16 to consent – see 11.7 for details on the Gillick case.

A child is deemed Gillick competent if they can understand, retain, use and weigh the information given and if they understand benefits, risks and consequences.

Involving the parents

Even if a child is competent enough to make a decision to consent to a given procedure or treatment, you should make every effort to encourage the child to involve their parents. Whatever their involvement, parents cannot override consent given by a competent child. If the child is not Gillick competent, authority to treat may be given by someone with parental responsibility under the Children Act 1989. Parental responsibility is assumed by:

- Both the child's natural parents, if they were married at the time of the birth or married later
- The father, if named on the birth certificate, if the child was born on or after 1 December 2003
- Step-parents can acquire parental responsibility in certain circumstances

Can children refuse treatment?

In Scotland the situation is simple. Children can refuse treatment and the child's decision cannot be overridden by the parents. Interestingly, parental responsibility for births registered in Scotland rests with:

- The father, if married to the mother when the child was conceived or married to the mother at any point afterwards
- An unmarried father, if named on the child's birth certificate, if the child was born after 4 May 2006

In England, Wales and Northern Ireland, no minor can refuse consent to treatment, when consent has been given by someone with parental responsibility or by the court. This applies even if the child is competent and specifically refuses treatment that is considered to be in their best interest. This is a rare event and you should seek legal advice through your trust and your defence union. Enforcing treatment on a child against their will poses risks, which need to be weighed up against the benefits of the procedure or treatment. You will also undoubtedly need to involve other members of the multidisciplinary team and an independent advocate for the child.

The above is the essential information, which you will be required to know for most interviews. If you are applying for paediatric dentistry, the policy document produced on behalf of the British Society of Paediatric Dentistry in 2008 is worth reviewing (Nunn J, et al. British Society of Paediatric Dentistry: a policy document on consent and the use of physical intervention in the dental care of children[19]).

---

[19] *Int J Paediatr Dent* 2008;18(Suppl 1):39–46).

11.7   Gillick competence and Fraser guidelines

In specialties where children are involved, questions are sometimes asked that require some basic knowledge of Gillick competence and Fraser guidelines.

These two concepts both relate to the ability of children to give consent for treatment, without the need for parental consent or knowledge. However, many candidates misunderstand or confuse the two concepts. In reality, although linked, they are slightly different. The purpose of this section is to explain what they mean and how they differ.

Gillick competence – The House of Lords ruling

In 1980 the Department of Health and Social Services (DHSS) advised doctors that children under the age of 16 could be prescribed contraception, without parental consent.

Mrs Gillick, the mother of ten children, including five daughters, sought a declaration from the House of Lords that the DHSS guidance was unlawful and adversely affected parental rights and duties. Her main arguments were that the decision was the same as administering treatment to a child without consent (which should rest with the parents), and that this encouraged others to commit the offence of having sexual relationships with a minor. Although she had won 3:0 in the Court of Appeal, she lost 2:3 in the House of Lords.

In 1985, the House of Lords panel, led by Lord Fraser, ruled that, if a minor was competent, parental rights did not exist and that the minor could consent to treatment without the parents being able to veto that decision. It was also ruled that the test of competence for minors should be the same as the test for competence for adults. This is now referred to as "Gillick competence". Although the Gillick case was originally solely about contraception, the ruling was general and applies to any treatment, investigation or procedure.

Further ruling

In 1990, a further ruling stated that a "Gillick-competent" child can prevent their parents from viewing their medical records. Consent must be sought explicitly.

Fraser guidelines

Following on from the Gillick case, Lord Fraser released further guidelines relating specifically to contraception (which can also be extended to abortion).

These guidelines state that a doctor or other health professional providing contraceptive advice or treatment to someone under 16, without parental consent, should be satisfied that all the following apply:

- The young person will understand the advice
- The young person will understand the moral, social and emotional implications
- The young person cannot be persuaded to tell their parents or allow the doctor to tell them that they are seeking contraceptive advice
- The young person is having, or is likely to have, unprotected sex, whether they receive the advice or not
- Their physical or mental health is likely to suffer unless they receive the advice or treatment
- It is in the young person's best interests to give contraceptive advice or treatment without parental consent

The relevance for dentistry lies in the implications of Gillick/Fraser competence in consenting to treatment, as the principles are extrapolated to other areas of healthcare.

A good overview of consent principles for children and young people generally is available online.[20]

---

[20] https://www.nhs.uk/conditions/consent-to-treatment/children/

11.8 Mental Capacity Act 2005 (effective 2007)

Although no in-depth knowledge of the Mental Capacity Act 2005 is required, candidates will be expected to know its key points. Many of the Mental Capacity Act 2005's provisions have been described in previous sections on consent. This section summarises the key components of the act.

Purpose of the act

The act formalises best practice and common law principles, in relation to the care of patients who lack capacity, and those who make decisions on their behalf.

Assessing lack of capacity

- No one can be assumed to lack capacity simply because they have a specific medical condition.

- Lack of capacity cannot be established in relation to someone's age, appearance or behaviour, which may lead others to make assumptions. So, for example:
  - Children are not necessarily lacking capacity simply because they are young.
  - Someone who is unkempt does not necessarily lack capacity simply because they are not looking after themselves.
  - Someone behaving eccentrically or making decisions that appear unusual or counter-intuitive does not necessarily lack capacity.

- Any action or decision taken on behalf of someone who lacks capacity must be taken in their best interest. Best interest can be assessed by asking the patient to write their wishes down (e.g. advanced directive) and by consulting those who are familiar with the patient (e.g. relatives or carers).

- Anyone providing care to a person who lacks capacity can do so without the risk of incurring legal liability, provided that capacity has been properly assessed and that care is being provided in line with the patient's best interest.

- The use or threat of force (called "restraint") is permitted only if the person using it believes that it will prevent harm to the patient who lacks capacity. With regard to the concept of "clinical holding", paediatric dentistry applicants in particular are directed to relevant guidance from the British Society of Paediatric Dentistry (BSPD).[21]

---

[21]https://www.bspd.co.uk/Portals/0/BSPD%20clinical%20holding%20guidelines%20final%20with%20flow%20chart%2020250416.pdf

Making decisions on behalf of an incapable patient and legal framework

- A patient with capacity is allowed to appoint an attorney to make health and welfare decisions on their behalf, should they ever lose capacity. This is called "Lasting Powers of Attorney" (LPA).

- Deputies may be appointed by the Court of Protection (COP) to make decisions in relation to welfare, healthcare and finances, though they cannot refuse consent to life-sustaining treatment. These court-appointed deputies will be supervised by the Office of the Public Guardian (OPG), established in 2007.

Protecting vulnerable people

- If a patient lacks capacity, but has no one to speak on their behalf, then an independent mental capacity advocate (IMCA) can be appointed to represent them. The IMCA cannot make decisions but represents the patient by bringing to the attention of decision makers the important factors that need to be considered, such as the patient's beliefs, feelings and values. The IMCA can also challenge decisions on behalf of the patient.

- Advanced decisions to refuse treatment: patients may provide an advanced statement that they refuse to receive treatment should they lose capacity in the future. The act states that the advanced decision can only be valid if a proper process has been followed. In particular, the statement must be in writing, signed and witnessed. For an advanced statement to be valid in cases of life-threatening events, the document must state explicitly that it is valid "even if life is at risk".

Using patients lacking capacity in research (this section would be relevant for those applying to academic posts)

- Any research involving patients lacking capacity should be approved by a research ethics committee (REC) and the intention to involve those patients made explicit at the time of requesting REC review. One condition is that there is no other alternative, i.e. that the research cannot be carried out using patients who have capacity instead.

- Approval should be sought from carers or nominated third parties before the patient can participate in the research. In particular, they should make a judgement as to whether the patient would have wanted to be involved.

If the patient concerned refuses to be involved or shows any sign of resistance, then they should not be included.

11.9 Consent when dealing with emergencies in the clinical setting

If you are dealing with emergencies in the clinical setting, then all the rules described in previous sections apply.

If a patient is competent at that time and needs a procedure, you should seek consent, even if only verbal.

If the patient is not competent and you cannot determine the patient's wishes through the relatives or other sources, then you can treat them without their consent, on the condition that the treatment that you administer is limited to what is immediately necessary to save their life or prevent a serious deterioration of their condition. The guidelines also specify that the treatment you provide must be the least restrictive of the patient's future choices. If the patient regains capacity, you should explain what was done. For any other treatment beyond the strict minimum, you should seek consent from the patient.

This is unlikely to feature heavily in dental interviews but may be a consideration in scenarios at dental core trainee (DCT) recruitment, to posts rotating through oral and maxillofacial surgery.

The GDC recommends that all registrants follow the guidance on medical emergencies management and training updates provided by Resuscitation Council UK and its main medical guidance, *Quality standards for cardiopulmonary resuscitation and training.*[22]

---

[22] https://www.resus.org.uk/quality-standards/

11.10 Reading list

For the most part, issues of consent and confidentiality are often common sense. There is little that you actually need to memorise once you have read this chapter, and understood how these concepts interact and how they may apply in your clinical practice.

In an interview, when questions are asked that relate to consent and confidentiality, the interviewers will expect you to demonstrate a degree of confidence and fluency. They will also expect you to demonstrate that you can involve the appropriate colleagues and other sources of help if you do not know the answer to the question. The information contained in this chapter will be more than enough for any interview at DCT or ST level.

Available from the General Dental Council (GDC)

- *Standards for the Dental Team*, particularly Principle 3, which deals specifically with obtaining valid consent.[23]

Available from the Office of Public Sector Information

- Mental Capacity Act 2005[24]

  This document is complex to read (legal jargon and with a formal legal format), so we would recommend that you read it only if you have an interest in these issues and a few hours to spare! Otherwise, the summary provided in section 11.8 will be more than enough.

Available from the specialist societies

- The British Orthodontic Society document *Professional Standards for Orthodontic Practice*[25]
- British Society for Paediatric Dentistry 2011 document *Guidelines for the Management of Children Referred for Dental Extractions Under General Anaesthesia*[26]

---

[23]https://standards.gdc-uk.org/pages/principle3/principle3.aspx
[24]www.opsi.gov.uk/ACTS/acts2005/ukpga_20050009_en_1
[25]https://www.bos.org.uk/Portals/0/Public/docs/Advice%20Sheets/Orthodontic%20Standards%20Document%20Final.pdf
[26]http://dentalanaesthesia.org.uk/wp-content/uploads/2016/08/full_guidelines_dopd_ga-1.pdf

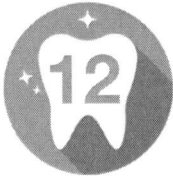

12 Difficult scenarios

Questions relating to confidentiality, consent or other ethical issues can be asked at interviews in any specialties.

Cascading questions

When ethical, consent and confidentiality issues are tested in the form of verbal interview questions (as opposed to role play), they tend to be asked in a cascading fashion, i.e. you are asked a simple initial question and, as soon as you provide an answer, the interviewers tell you that your approach is not working and add extra information to make the problem more complex.

For example, you explain that you deal with a problem by seeking help from a registrar; the interviewers will tell you that he is not available. You then state that you would contact the consultant. The interviewers tell you that he is not answering his phone; and so on. The best way you can deal with them is by:

* Remaining calm and remembering that these questions are not designed to make you fail but to test your understanding of the issues involved
* Making sure that you do not simply explain what you would do, but how you arrive at that conclusion, i.e. what is driving your actions, explaining the ethical principles that you use whenever appropriate
* Reassuring yourself that what is important is your thinking process, so make sure that you set out the logic of your arguments

Once you have learnt to deal with a few key scenarios, then you can pretty much deal with any scenario that is thrown at you. Therefore, instead of learning all possible scenarios by heart, make sure that you understand the basic concepts that underpin the management of each situation. The theory set out in Section 11 and the examples that follow should help you with this.

12.1 Maxillofacial surgery: You have a 20-year-old patient on the ward. She has told you that she does not get on with her father and that, if he calls, you should not tell him anything about her condition. Later on that day, one of the nurses tells you that the father is on the phone, aggressively demanding some information. What do you do?

The ethics

In normal circumstances, most patients would authorise you to provide information to their relatives. In this case, however, the patient has explicitly told you that she did not want her father to be told anything and therefore you have to respect her wishes.

The fact that the patient is 20 years old is in fact a red herring, because the same principle would apply to a 14-year-old. In principle, every patient is entitled to confidentiality unless you have a good reason to breach it.

The communication

From an ethical point of view, the answer is almost too simple. What the interviewers will therefore be more interested in is the way in which you handle the matter. There are dozens of ways in which this can be achieved. Here are some:

- Ask the nurse to reassure the father that someone will be with him soon. If it may be some time, the father should be told that someone will call back shortly.
- Use the time to discuss with the daughter whether she stands by her decision. You may want to enquire as to the reasons behind her refusal, to see if there is an easy way of breaking the deadlock. You should not push too far (you don't want to be involved too much in their family feuds).
- See if you can try to reach a compromise. For example, if the patient is not in any danger, she may agree to her father being told that she is fine so that he is reassured (after all, he may not be concerned about the detail of the problem and may simply want to know that his daughter is safe).
- Take the phone call (or call the father back) and introduce yourself.
- Provide the father with whatever information was agreed with the patient. If the patient asked you to say nothing at all, then you will need to explain this to the father sensitively.
- Recommend that the father talks to his daughter directly.

266

- If the father insists or becomes more aggressive, explain that you will discuss the matter with a senior colleague and end the call, after the usual civilities.
- Discuss the matter with a consultant.

Probing: Still unhappy, the father turns up on the ward that afternoon demanding an explanation. He is abusive towards members of staff. What do you do?

Your priority will be the safety of the staff, the patient and the other patients. You and suitable staff members should take the father away from the ward. If he causes problems, you should call the security team.

Once the father has been isolated, you should make sure that no one is on their own with him. Take a colleague with you and talk to him about the situation. The father should be reminded that his behaviour is not acceptable, after which you should determine what his causes for worry are.

Similar principles to the telephone conversation will apply from then on, i.e. you can only reveal information that the patient has agreed for you to disclose. If the father wants to know more, then you should encourage him to discuss the matter with his daughter.

When the father has left, you may want to discuss the matter further with the daughter to see if you can break the deadlock.

12.2 Oral surgery: You are supervising a busy MOS/GA session and a junior has inadvertently extracted the wrong tooth (LR5 instead of LR4). How do you deal with this event?

The first thing to establish is exactly:

1. What were the indications for the extraction, e.g. orthodontic extraction
2. When can one dental unit be substituted for another (subject to discussion with the referring orthodontist)?
3. Establish whether what the trainee thinks has happened has actually taken place
4. Establish what the patient has been told, before approaching them to explain what is, in effect, a never event.

Remember, you are a trainee. Whilst you are a middle grade and have a duty of clinical care to the patient, and pastoral care to the trainee who is your junior, you also follow a chain of command to your consultant / educational supervisor. They will need to be informed early on and senior help/support involved.

- Approach the patient and explain clearly what has happened, making sure that post-operative measures have been instituted, as for any extraction; whilst at the same time ensuring that the tooth is stored in an appropriate medium, pending a senior opinion.
- Start contacting your consultant in order to make a plan.

Probing: The consultant in oral surgery who is responsible for the patient, and due to be supervising the clinic, is unavailable and cannot be reached.

Answer:
- Call another consultant. Potentially, if these are orthodontic extractions, consider calling a consultant orthodontist, ideally the orthodontist who has made the treatment plan, but any senior orthodontic opinion will be valuable in making a time-critical decision.

Probing: There is no orthodontist available to give an opinion.

Remember the basic tenet of *primum non nocere*, or "first do no harm". Clearly, in this rather improbable situation, the basic principles are:

- Do not continue with the treatment, e.g. the other planned extractions.
- Strongly consider replanting the extracted tooth. This may be the best way to leave all options open for further treatment decisions.
- Arrange the next available appointment with your consultant in oral surgery and the referring consultant orthodontist, ideally jointly.
- Be candid and honest with the patient and their relatives about what has happened.

The "least unsafe" principle

The interviewers are constantly placing hurdles in your way to make situations as unsafe as they can and to force you into make an unwise decision – a common theme in these types of scenario. In this scenario, none of the safe options are available to you and you must therefore opt for the least unsafe solution.

As stated, the important thing is to be open, candid, honest and transparent, and to think about the least irreversible management decision to make the best of a bad situation.

Risk management

Once the situation is over, you must then deal with the other issues. In this scenario there are a few issues that need to be addressed with the team:

- Completion of an incident form
- Ascertaining institutional learning
- Presentation of the incident at a clinical governance or morbidity meeting
- Ensuring that steps are taken to make sure this is not repeated, e.g. reviewing the checklist procedure for "counting down" teeth
- Whether a root cause analysis (RCA) is warranted, to ascertain what happened on this occasion, as well as why there were issues contacting senior personnel

Last but not least, consider the more junior trainee. Remember that, as a middle grade, you are the leader of tomorrow, and as such, you are cultivating your future as a trainer. The trainee who is junior to you in this scenario may well be completely devastated about what has happened and require as much support as they can get. Spend time with them, offer to walk through what happened together, encourage a reflective report from them (which is good practice but can also be cathartic) and offer to accompany them to any meeting with their educational supervisor or RCA review board.

12.3 Maxillofacial surgery: You are a DCT on call for the maxillofacial team, and a patient is brought in with stridor and impending airway compromise from Ludwig's angina. Outline how you would assess and manage the patient.

The key is your level of training, which is very junior. Your aim here is to be safe, keep seniors in the loop, and make the situation as controlled as possible by being a lynchpin for all the people who are going to get involved in helping this patient. The ability to prioritise, delegate, pass information up the chain and operate within (and sometimes just beyond) your comfort zone are all key features of this scenario.

Remember not to get too bogged down in the clinical detail. As with other interview stations, within reason, these elements are not overly of interest. Interpersonal relationships, communication skills, ethical decision making and professionalism are amongst the attributes being examined here.

Answer:

- Think ahead and if, possible, ask for observations and basic measures to be instituted before you arrive.
- Let your registrar and/or consultant know where you are going and what you are going to see – their ears may well prick up!
- Make an initial assessment of the patient.
- Institute appropriate initial measures, e.g. 15 L/min oxygen through non-rebreathe mask, intravenous (IV) access, airway adjuncts.
- Delegate tasks if possible, e.g. sending bloods, contacting help.
- Often in such scenarios the help available to you is limited in terms of people and skill mix, e.g. one healthcare assistant (HCA) or inexperienced nurse.
- Contact help from your middle grade and/or begin readying theatres and contacting the on-call anaesthetist.
- Move the patient to a resuscitation bay in the emergency department.
- See if anyone within the department has advanced airway skills.

Probing: Help is not forthcoming as everyone is tied up elsewhere, and the patient begins to take a turn for the worse, encountering obvious difficulty breathing, with dropping oxygen saturations.

Answer:

- Revisit everything you have done so far; remember, many of these answers are about being systematic and demonstrating "mirror, signal and manoeuvre" approaches to answering.
- Could you have used any airway adjuncts or similar, e.g. Guedel, nasopharyngeal?
- Revisit the idea of enlisting help from anyone available, e.g. someone in ED with advanced airway skills.

Probing: *A junior anaesthetist attends to review the patient, and at this moment, the patient loses their airway and their oxygen saturations plummet. The anaesthetist makes attempts to intubate the patient but fails and is unable to establish an airway.*

This is now way outside of your comfort zone. We would stress that this is an example of how to think in these questions, but essentially you want to do something that is the "least unsafe", as highlighted in the previous example. Clearly, this is a rather contrived scenario, but under the circumstances you cannot *do nothing*. Therefore, an invasive airway of some sort is warranted.

Guidelines such as those from the Difficult Airway Society (das.uk.com) are clear in a "can't intubate, can't ventilate" situation, that every measure should be tried first, such as head extension, jaw thrusts, oral/nasal airway adjuncts. A laryngeal mask airway (LMA™), with maximum two attempts permitted, comes next. The key here is that a person trained in advanced airway skills has tried to intubate the patient via the standard approach and failed,

In our opinion, a needle cricothyroidotomy is the safest option here, as:

- It is the lowest-risk front-of-neck airway access manoeuvre
- You potentially can do very little to worsen the situation and, at the very least, stabilise things for a brief period of time (insufflating oxygen, but not ventilating the patient) until senior help arrives
- You are faced with no alternative but to do something you have read about or been told about on a DCT trauma skills course, but remember that many of your consultants will not have placed a needle cricothyroidotomy! It is making the best of a *very* bad situation and is likely to be something you never, ever have to do in your career. Ever.

Again, we would stress that this is a patient in *extremis*, which you are unlikely to encounter in your clinical practice as a well-supported DCT in the NHS. However, the principle of stretching outside your comfort zone, to do the "least unsafe" thing for the patient, is the learning point in answering these questions.

12.4 Special care dentistry: A patient with learning difficulties is brought into the clinic requiring an extraction. During the procedure, the patient's mother faints and becomes unresponsive. What do you do?

This scenario plays on a number of points, including your ability to prioritise, delegate, deal with a potential medical emergency and seek support early. You have essentially progressed from having one patient to now having two patients, and you are midway through a procedure, with the patient in the chair, and have no clinical history of the "patient" who is now on the floor!

Answer:

- You need to ascertain where you are in your patient's management. Is this a safe point where you can suspend treatment, e.g. has the extraction not yet commenced, concluded?
- You need to work out what resources you have to hand, e.g. who is around you currently, who can you get help from in the setting you are in, and do you have emergency drugs and/or defibrillator if required?
- Could the patient help you with a collateral history concerning the mother and any medications/conditions she may have? Do not presume a vasovagal – whilst the simplest explanation is the most likely, there are more serious explanations that, whilst uncommon, cannot be missed!

Probing: You have a dental nurse with you, who is scrubbed for the procedure and a second acting as a "runner". You are in a community setting with no on-site "crash" team.

Answer:

- Delegate the nurse to look after the patient. You need to prioritise, and in this situation, in the current format, the mother is the sicker of the two people, with a degree of uncertainty concerning just how serious her situation is. Arguably, this is likely to be a vasovagal syncope, but the worst-case scenario should be catered for.
- You need to make sure the mother is in a position of safety and that basic life support (BLS) measures begin, with resuscitation if required, and application of defibrillator pads if needed.
- CALL FOR HELP EARLY, or delegate the runner to do so. In a community setting, this will mean a 999 call early in the scenario.

- In the meantime, the nurse should continue to stay with the patient, unless able to be freed up to help you, in which case you can delegate jobs such as setting up oxygen to give to the mother, as part of BLS.
- As always, the detail is largely irrelevant in a simulated scenario for the purposes of an interview, but the ability to prioritise and delegate effectively when under pressure is more keenly examined.

The General Dental Council is clear in stating that "all registrants must be trained in dealing with medical emergencies, including resuscitation, and possess up to date evidence of capability".

Furthermore, the Care Quality Commission (CQC) states that, in line with Resuscitation Council UK quality standards, the following is the *minimum* equipment requirement for a dental surgery setting:

- Adhesive defibrillator pads
- Automated external defibrillator (AED)
- Face masks for self-inflating bag
- Oropharyngeal airways
- Oxygen cylinder
- Oxygen masks with reservoir
- Oxygen tubing
- Pocket mask with oxygen port
- Portable suction
- Protective equipment
- Razor
- Scissors
- Self-inflating bag with reservoir (adult and child versions)

Probing: The patient tells you that his mother is a diabetic and that her medication is in her bag. You look in her bag and find a device to self-administer insulin. What do you do?

Remember that you are being pushed out of your comfort zone. You do not have enough information to hand to make a decision about whether this would be safe (and in all likelihood, the mother may well be hypoglycaemic – administering insulin could prove to fatal!). Technically, she is also not your patient, so there are issues surrounding that consideration. The GDC advises registrants to act with integrity and maintain public trust in the profession, and defence unions such as the Dental Defence Union[27] may provide indemnity for claims arising from good-Samaritan acts carried out anywhere. Arguably therefore, the right thing to do, being the most

---

[27]https://www.theddu.com/my-membership/member-guide/ddu-member-guide/defending-you

qualified person available, is to offer support and help, commensurate with your level of training.

Your role is to institute BLS measures as required and keep the patient safe, whilst getting appropriate help. If you are able to ascertain a capillary blood-glucose level, using a point-of-care device, and can establish that the mother is hypoglycaemic, it may be safe to administer oral glucose (if the patient is rousable/conscious) or IM glucagon.

The CQC states that, in line with NICE guidance on prescribing in dental practice for medical emergencies, the following drugs should be available within the practice:

- Adrenaline 1mg/ml
- Aspirin dispersible tablets 300mg
- Glucagon 1unit vial
- Glucose (for administration by mouth)
- Glyceryl trinitrate spray
- Midazolam oral mucosal solution
- Oxygen
- Salbutamol 100 micrograms / metered inhalation

An excellent trainee will look for "final flourishes" in answering any question, such as:

- The possibility of institutional learning through a team debrief and/or clinical governance meeting
- Ensuring everyone felt well supported and was up to date with resuscitation training
- Possibly arranging a simulated session, to institute lasting positive change within a department/practice
- Considering writing a reflective report
- Seeking feedback from the events in the form of a work-based assessment (WBA) or similar
- Maybe a timely revisit of the management of medical emergencies in dental practice / surgery settings for a publication!

12.5 Paediatric dentistry: A 12-year-old boy attends for a dental emergency treatment session with his uncle, and you notice advanced caries and note that he is an infrequent attendee, who only attends sporadically with infections. What do you do?

- The boy is 12 years old. According to the Gillick competence principle and Fraser guidelines, if he is competent, then he would be able to consent to emergency dental treatment. Every effort should, however, be made to contact those who have "parental responsibility" for the child (parents/guardians) and ensure that they are happy with this treatment, or defer treatment where possible.

- The uncle cannot consent for the child and the law is clear on this matter. Treatment on this occasion should be confined to emergency treatment. People other than those with parental responsibility can make decisions within confined parameters if authorised to do so by the parents/guardians.

- The peripheral issue is that of "dental neglect". The British Society of Paediatric Dentistry has highlighted in a policy document on dental neglect, published in the *International Journal of Paediatric Dentistry* in 2009, that dental neglect can be defined as "the persistent failure to meet a child's basic oral health needs, likely to result in the serious impairment of a child's oral or general health or development".

- This is a label applied not with regard to the severity/extent of dental caries *per se* in isolation, but when taken in context with other dental and non-dental factors, such as past dental attendance records, severity and duration of symptoms and any adverse events (e.g. multiple general anaesthesia session for dental extractions, episodes of severe dental infection). Non-dental signs of neglect should be sought, as highlighted in Harris J et al. *Child Protection and the Dental Team: An Introduction to Safeguarding Children in Dental Practice.* Sheffield: Committee of Postgraduate Dental Deans and Directors, 2006.[28]

- Identification of dental neglect should prompt preventive dental team management, preventive multi-agency management and a child protection referral. Thus, you are looking beyond the face-value issues of consent and thinking more broadly, including giving due deference to multidisciplinary working and holistic care of children.

---

[28] http://www.cpdt.org.uk

- There should be a recognition of the need to work with the family and bring the parents in to the consultations going forwards, shifting the emphasis from blame to support, with realistic treatment planning to ensure attendance.

- Other professionals involved in the child's care may need to be contacted and involved, such as the school nurse, doctor, or social worker, to establish a joint plan of action and make the welfare of the child the priority, ideally informing those with parental responsibility and the child in question beforehand, if possible.

- Local protection procedures should be followed if there are concerns about ongoing dental neglect or other signs of neglect or abuse, and dentists need to recognise that they may be called upon to provide evidence in child-protection cases for this very reason.

12.6 Generic: You are a dental specialty trainee in <xxx>. A young female trainee dentist refuses to deal with a patient who is a known rapist. What do you do?

In such questions it is very easy to jump to conclusions and to assume that the trainee is in breach of her duties by not giving the patient the care he is entitled to. However, the situation may be more complex than it first appears.

You can answer this question using the SPIES structure set out in section 5.3.

Seek information
Although you would want to find out more about the reasons behind the trainee's decision, the time for discussion will come later, once the immediate issue of patient care/safety has been dealt with.

Patient care/safety
The patient is entitled to care, regardless of his background, and you must ensure that it is delivered by someone whose behaviour is not being affected by their beliefs.

There may be several reasons for the trainee to refuse to see the patient, and this will need to be investigated. Whether she feels threatened in any way, or whether it is simply on principle, she is not best placed to treat this patient (after all, there is no point forcing her). Therefore, you may want to manage the patient yourself or to delegate the responsibility to someone who is more willing.

Initiative
Once the patient's problem has been resolved, you ought to organise a discussion with the junior trainee to get to the bottom of the issue, as her behaviour may have consequences on the future delivery of patient care, particularly if there are other types of patients that she finds it difficult to deal with. You will want to identify why she refused to manage the patient.

- Perhaps she or someone close to her was raped in the past. If this were the case, she may feel physically threatened (even if there was no explicit threat from the patient) and would not be safe in dealing with the patient.
- Perhaps the patient actually made some remarks towards her, in which case she might have felt physically threatened.
- Perhaps she is simply prejudiced and is making a point of principle. If this were the case, she would likely be in breach of her duties as a dentist, which requires that dentists should not let their personal beliefs interfere with the care of patients (GDC *Standards* Principle 1: Put patient's interests first).

If the trainee had felt threatened, then she would need support from a senior colleague to overcome such fears and agree a strategy, should the problem occur again.

If the trainee showed signs of prejudice, then you would need to remind her of her duties and would also need to report the matter to a senior colleague so that they can discuss the situation with her.

Escalate

Either way, this looks like a serious situation, which could have serious effects on the trainee's mental wellbeing. Whether there has been a breach of duty or not, it would make sense to encourage the trainee to discuss the matter with a senior colleague, and, if this does not happen, to raise the matter yourself, albeit informally.

There is also a chance that the patient may make a complaint, and it would make sense for senior colleagues to be made aware of the problem before the patient himself escalated it.

Support

Whichever way you look at the situation, the trainee has clearly been affected by the matter, and you owe her a degree of support. If there were a number of members of staff affected by this patient or incident, it may be worth organising a team debrief, facilitated by an appropriate professional, such as a psychologist.

12.7 Generic: You find out that one of your consultants is romantically involved with someone who is a current patient of the department. What do you do?

This question is difficult because, although we are told that the patient is a current patient of the department, it is not clear whether that patient is being treated by that consultant. It is possible that the consultant in question told their partner to get referred to their own department because they have faith in the quality of the service being delivered there, thinking it would be fine if they are not themselves seeing their own partner in clinic.

The whole answer rests on the notion of whether this would seem appropriate or not, and this is not always clear-cut.

Scenario 1: The consultant is treating the patient (or involved in some way in the patient's care)

This situation is inappropriate. If the relationship started before the partner became a patient, then he/she should not be treated by the consultant, as the potential for the consultant to remain objective and impartial is conceivably impaired. If the relationship started when the partner was already a patient, then this is even more improper.

The matter should be reported to the consultant's line manager (i.e. the clinical director), and the GDC would then likely need to be notified. In essence, the behaviour exhibited, particularly in taking advantage of a current dentist–patient relationship to commence a romantic relationship, is in contravention of GDC *Standard* 9.1 "You must ensure that your conduct, both at work and in your personal life, justifies patients' trust in you and the public's trust in the dental profession."

Scenario 2: The consultant is not treating the patient (or involved in any way in the patient's care)

This situation is a bit more complicated because there is no established dentist-patient relationship as such. However, there are grounds to argue that this can be contentious. For example:

* The consultant has easy access to the partner's clinical records.
* The consultant may come across details of the partner's medical/dental condition.
* The consultant may influence their colleagues on choice of treatment.

In the interest of transparency, the consultant should be advised to declare their relationship with the patient to their manager (i.e. the clinical director), so that the situation can be discussed and a conclusion can be reached. In such situations, it is unlikely that the GDC will be involved, but safeguards may be introduced to ensure complete separation between the consultant and the partner's clinical records.

In particular, accessing health records of partners, relatives and friends without good justifiable reasons have led to a number of NHS staff being suspended, having employment terminated and/or being referred to their respective regulatory bodies. Such health-record access has monetary implications for the employing organisation, with the Information Commissioner's Office (ICO) having the power to impose monetary penalties of up to £500,000 on data controllers for violation of General Data Protection Regulation (GDPR) and the Data Protection Act 2018.

What the GDC says

GDC *Standard* 9.1.4 states "You must maintain appropriate boundaries in the relationships you have with patients. You must not take advantage of your position as a dental professional in your relationships with patients."

Equally, in GDC guidance on prescribing, registrants are asked to prescribe "only when you are able to form an objective view of your patient's health and clinical needs". A lack of objectivity may mean missing crucial information and/or impaired judgement and decision-making that would be outwith your normal standards.

Current patients

In ending a professional relationship with a patient, you are essentially adhering to GDC *Standard* 1.7.8, which states that "Before you end a professional relationship with a patient, you must be satisfied that your decision is fair and you must be able to justify your decision. You should write to the patient to tell them your decision and your reasons for it. You should take steps to ensure that arrangements are made promptly for the continuing care of the patient."

Former patients

Personal relationships with former patients may also be inappropriate, depending on factors such as:

- The length of time since the professional relationship ended (the more recently a professional relationship with a patient ended, the less likely it is that beginning a personal relationship with that patient would be appropriate)

- The nature of the previous professional relationship

- Whether the patient was particularly vulnerable at the time of the professional relationship, and whether they are still vulnerable

- Whether you will be caring for other members of the patient's family

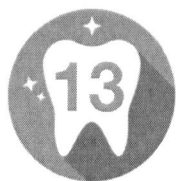

13 NHS issues and hot topics

Most candidates have limited knowledge of NHS structures and policy; as a result, many worry that they could face difficult factual questions, which they would be unable to answer. These are uncommon (if asked at all) at dental core training and specialty training interviews, and are more commonplace at consultant interviews. However, they can conceivably make an appearance at recruitment to specialities such as dental public health.

On the whole, questions on NHS issues are designed to test your general understanding of the issues rather than detailed knowledge of any particular topic. In other words, you are more likely to be asked "How do you feel the specialty will be affected by current NHS changes?" than "Tell us everything you know about the Darzi report". You should therefore make some effort to familiarise yourself with key issues likely to affect the specialty to which you are applying, and reflect on their significance to your career and your specialty. By demonstrating a good understanding of these issues, you will present yourself as a mature candidate with strong motivation.

Different types of questions

NHS issues can be tested at interview in three main ways:

- Knowledge questions about a specific topic, e.g. "What is the role of the Care Quality Commission?"

- Awareness questions such as "What do you think about the increasing role of the private sector?"

- Application questions, i.e. questions that require putting together a range of ideas such as "What are the issues affecting this specialty at the moment?", or "How do you see this specialty evolving over the next 5 or 10 years?"

As well as being tested through standard interview questions, your knowledge of NHS issues can be tested through presentations and group discussions.

What the interviewers are looking for

The interviewers will be looking for three features:

- The effort that you have put into keeping abreast of current developments relevant to your specialty, and therefore your motivation for the specialty

- Your ability to analyse the impact of these issues on your work environment and the health system in general, and therefore your debating ability and general level of maturity

- Your ability to communicate your ideas in a structured and convincing fashion

Specialty-specific NHS issues and hot topics

In some interviews, you may be asked about specific documents or issues relating to your specialty. This could include NHS England's Guides for Commissioning Dental Specialties, specific NICE or other guidelines, or the place of managed clinical networks (MCNs) and/or local dental networks (LDNs). To ensure that you can answer all these questions, you should consult the following sources of information:

- The NHS England guidance on dental commissioning[29]
- The NICE website
- The relevant royal-college websites
- Specialist society websites
- Information available from your LDN and associated specialty-specific MCN
- NHS England guidance on LDNs[30]
- Up-and-coming issues related to dentistry, in particular contracts and commissioning from the popular press, e.g. BBC News[31]

You should ask some of your senior colleagues to point you in the direction of specialty-specific issues and guidelines that are topical at the time of your interview. You should also read specialty-specific papers, as interviewers sometimes ask questions on papers that have recently been published.

---

[29] https://www.england.nhs.uk/primary-care/dentistry/dental-commissioning/
[30] https://www.england.nhs.uk/primary-care/dentistry/leading-the-change/local-dental-networks/
[31] https://www.bbc.co.uk/news/health

General NHS issues and hot topics

These are general topics that apply to most specialties. This includes issues such as the current NHS drive towards better quality and more efficiency, the issues of patient choice and increased competition, or issues relating to the impact of current reforms on dental training. It is crucial that you understand the key messages and are able to present your own opinion of the possible impact on the department to which you are applying. It is important to be aware that most reports have a brief executive summary, which gives the highlights and is easier to digest if you're short of time.

A sensible word of advice

In the whole scheme of things, questions on NHS issues do not get asked at many interviews.

In the course of your preparation, although it is important that you gain an overview of current issues, beware not to get bogged down with insignificant detail, as this is never probed into. All that will be required of you is an overall understanding of these issues; the summaries that follow will be more than enough to help you achieve the required level of understanding.

We would advise strongly that you allocate the majority of your preparation time to all the other types of questions addressed in previous chapters, particularly if you are short of time.

13.1 Overview of the NHS in England

Commissioning of services

In England, each NHS trust essentially operates as an independent business. The decision as to which healthcare provider is allowed to provide which services is made by clinical commissioning groups (CCGs), which consist mainly of local GPs and managers (with a few representatives from hospitals).

Legislation that came into effect in 2013 has made it possible for external providers (e.g. charities or even private companies) to offer NHS services. So, for example, a local CCG could decide to award a contract for cataract surgery to a private company rather than to the local hospital (though of course they would need to have a good reason to do that – a good reason being that they feel the private company may provide better quality of care). The process of awarding contracts is known in the NHS as "commissioning".

Because CCGs are local groups and consist mainly of GPs, they cannot commission GP services themselves. Similarly, they can't commission services that need to be provided on a more global scale because of their specialist nature, such as heart and lung transplant surgery or eye cancer care, for two reasons:

1. They don't have the skills and knowledge to understand the exact nature of those services.

2. Those services are provided on a regional or national basis.

Instead, both primary care services and specialist services are commissioned by a higher body, which used to be called the NHS Commissioning Board but is now known simply as NHS England. They are also concerned with the commissioning of dental services – primary care and the dental specialties.

Differences in dentistry

NHS England commissions dental services including specialist, community and out-of-hours dental services. The *Introductory Guide for Commissioning Dental Specialties*[32] gives a good overview of the landscape of dental specialty commissioning.

---

[32]https://www.england.nhs.uk/commissioning/wp-content/uploads/sites/12/2015/09/intro-guide-comms-dent-specl.pdf

The key features common to all dental specialties are:

- The initial commissioning guide development covered oral surgery and oral medicine, orthodontics, special care dentistry and restorative dentistry.
- There are plans to follow these with paediatric dentistry, restorative monospecialties and supporting services, including dental and maxillofacial radiology, oral microbiology and oral Pathology.
- There has been an effort to achieve consistency across England in agreeing details such as referral criteria, core data-set requirements, contractual frameworks, and quality of environment and equipment.
- A framework is in place to ensure clinical engagement and forward planning, utilising specialty-specific managed clinical networks (MCNs) and local professional networks (LPNs) or local dental networks (LDNs) to optimise the patient journey from primary dental care to specialist services.
- This echoes the sentiment outlined in the *NHS Five Year Forward View* (2014), which stated "Increasingly we need to manage systems – networks of care – not just organisations".
- Procedural complexity is defined within dental specialties, to ensure that competencies are defined for clinicians providing specialist care. For instance, Level 1 complexity is that expected of someone who has completed a DFT programme. Level 2 requires enhanced skills and experience, but not necessarily specialist registration status, and such services may be provided within the community in nominated/accredited Level 2 provider contracts. Level 3 care is delivered by specialists/consultants in primary, dental hospital or secondary care, depending on patient and disease factors.

As an example, in oral surgery and oral medicine, there are difficulties faced by a heterogenous group of clinicians delivering services with different skillsets and interests: oral surgeons, oral and maxillofacial surgeons, and consultants and specialists in oral medicine. General dental practitioner (GDP) contribution to delivery of oral surgery and oral medicine can be variable, as can the proportion of dentists with special interests (DwSIs) serving a given population. Increasingly, particularly with regard to oral surgery, routine work is being "pushed" onto consultant waiting lists. In looking at the complexity of work, the levels can be defined on a procedural basis, for example:

- **Level 1:** Straightforward extraction
- **Level 2:** Surgical removal of uncomplicated third molars, exposure of buried teeth
- **Level 3:** Advanced implantology requiring bone grafting, enucleation of cysts, increased risk of iatrogenic nerve injury / antral involvement

In an "ideal" system, primary care practitioners would deliver Level 1 treatment, with accredited Level 2 providers delivering Level 2 treatments in primary care, with consultant-led assessment of competence and the same level of remuneration, regardless of the level of qualification of the clinician. Level 3 treatments would be provided by dental hospital / secondary / tertiary care specialists in oral surgery and/or oral and maxillofacial surgery.

Examples of good practice in this regard have included:

- Queensway Tees Oral Surgery Service (QTOSS) and Queensway Durham and Darlington Oral Surgery Service (QDDOSS), which have been lauded for being all specialist-run, with staff who are nationally accredited in sedation, running educational events for local DFTs and demonstrating a transparent and well-thought-out QA process
- Birmingham, where the MCN for oral surgery has representation from oral surgery, oral and maxillofacial surgery, general dental practitioners, commissioners and the salaried dental services, and where services are delivered by a "hub and spoke" model, with practices providing Level 2 oral surgery services in the community

Commissioning guides can be found on the NHS England website.[33]

Dentists in primary care provide treatment for the NHS under contracts – the general dental services (GDS) contract and the less common personal dental services (PDS) agreement.

To provide NHS dentistry, dentists require registration on the performers list, and remuneration is limited to specified "bands" of dental treatment of increasing treatment complexity, with associated units of dental activity (UDAs) and monetary values per UDA, based on individual earnings in a reference period. For instance, a Band 1 treatment might be a scale and polish and is associated with 1 UDA. From the inception of the UDA system, there was the suggestion that the number of complex treatments began to fall and dentists seemed to shift towards patterns of practice in an effort to hit UDA targets, as opposed to selecting on the basis of clinical considerations.

The contract system restricts the treatments on offer to patients, and alternatives may only be available on a private basis, with many practitioners therefore offering mixed private/NHS work in their practices. The system of UDAs was first introduced in 2006 and has come under some criticism as dentists are paid per course of treatment, regardless of how many items are provided within the said course of treatment (e.g. one filling would yield the same payment as five fillings, which would translate to 3 UDAs).

---

[33]https://www.england.nhs.uk/primary-care/dentistry/dental-commissioning/dental-specialities/

A review led by Professor Jimmy Steele and published in 2009 made suggestions for reconfiguration in the delivery of dental services; and in 2015 new dental prototypes were introduced, with plans for a new contract to be rolled out in April 2020, blending capitation and fee for service (FFS) models. "Blend A" models saw capitation covering Band 1 care only, with Bands 2 and 3 being subject to patient charges, whilst "Blend B" extended capitation to cover Band 1 and Band 2 care. The key consideration has been a shift of focus from treatment to prevention, with dental practices being remunerated for the number of patients they treat, and their quality of care rather than specific episodes of care.

13.2 The role of the private sector in the provision of healthcare in England

There are several ways in which the private sector is involved and, although you will not need to know any of this in much detail, you must know enough to understand which part of the private sector an interview question is referring to before you can answer it. The different types of private providers are as follows:

Private-practice doctors and dentists (referred to as "private healthcare")

This normally refers to clinicians working for private hospitals or for themselves, who provide healthcare to individual private patients. Examples of private healthcare providers include BUPA or AXA PPP. These private providers have been around for a long time and are normally used by patients to bypass the NHS waiting lists. Patients either pay for the care themselves or through a private healthcare insurance company. The clinicians involved in private healthcare are often the same as those working for the NHS, who undertake private activities in their spare time. The prices charged by those private providers are subject to market forces and are typically much higher than the standard NHS tariffs for the same procedures.

External (i.e. non-NHS) providers contracted to do NHS work

This refers to private companies, charities or other organisations who have been officially commissioned to provide healthcare to NHS patients at NHS tariffs. An example of this is Virgin Care, which provides services to NHS patients in areas as diverse as breast cancer screening, paediatric physiotherapy, sexual health services or dermatology clinics. Those services are commissioned by the CCGs, and are provided at no direct cost to the patient. Basically, this is NHS care provided at NHS tariffs by non-NHS providers. It is easy to see how Level 2 and/or 3 complexity work within dental specialties may similarly be commissioned by providers outside of the dental hospitals and/or secondary care facilities.

It is the introduction of those private providers, contracted to do NHS work, that has led many to fear a "privatisation of the NHS". Here are the arguments commonly presented for and against such a system (which we have tried to present in as balanced a way as possible):

- Private companies are run for profit. There is a risk that they will therefore favour making a profit over providing good-quality care. The counterargument to this is that the NHS has been run on a not-for-profit basis for many years and has not always provided the best-quality care it could (see, later, the section on the Mid-Staffordshire Trust). In addition, though there is some anecdotal evidence that some private companies engage in dubious practices or do not deliver in line with expectations, this is not widespread (and again the NHS has its own share of dubious practices too).

- Private companies may "cherry-pick" the easy cases that are the most profitable, leaving the NHS burdened with the more complex, loss-making cases. The answer to that argument is that it is, indeed, true, for the simple reason that one would not want those private companies to take on complex cases they can't handle. Those companies would be asked to handle the simple high-volume work to ensure that that work is being done efficiently without interference from other work such as emergencies; it follows, then, that the NHS (with more expertise than the private sector) should handle the more complex cases that it has been trained to handle well. The reason NHS trusts may be losing money on those more complex cases is because the tariffs have not been calculated well enough to ensure they can cover their costs. However, it is a matter of time before this anomaly is resolved.

- "Privatisation" would lead to fragmentation of care. If different aspects of care were given to different providers, then healthcare may be provided in many more venues than under the old system (where basically care was only provided either in a GP practice or in a hospital). This may mean that patients would have to travel to different places in order to be seen, which would cause issues with patient records, for example, since there is no central database that can be accessed from everywhere.

- The fragmentation of care described in the previous paragraph would also lead to training issues. External providers would be handling the simple cases, which are those used as part of training. A private company that needs to make a profit may be reluctant to train clinicians if that leads to a loss of profit.

- There are risks of conflict of interest amongst clinicians. Many of those external providers are, in fact, at least partially owned by healthcare professionals. Some hospital consultants have also set up external businesses, which could be competing against the same hospital trust in which they work. The commissioning of such services therefore has to be done in an open and transparent manner.

Many dentists in primary care will offer mixed NHS/private practices due to the restrictions in available treatment options available to patients on GDS contracts. Dental specialists may not infrequently deliver private care within dental practices where they may work as self-employed specialists on associate rates or enter into partnership, jointly owning the practice. Others may work in private hospitals, providing treatments to patients on a fee-paying basis or via private healthcare insurers. Clearly, with a restricted pool of dental specialists, sitting on the MCN and advising NHS England on commissioning services on the one hand, and owning a practice that possible delivers on Level 2 and/or 3 work, may easily become a conflict of interest. With the changes in commissioning for dental specialties, there may be opportunities for specialists and/or consultants to offer Level 2 work in particular by either entering into a direct contract with the commissioners (subject to ensuring standards) or being contracted to do NHS work by a trust with waiting-list issues.

13.3 The NHS Long Term Plan (2019)

Published on 7 January 2019, the NHS Long Term Plan (formerly known as the 10-year plan) was published, setting out key ambitions for the period 2019–2029. It builds on the previously published NHS Five Year Forward View, which articulated the needs to integrate care to meet the needs of a changing population. The main features of the NHS Long Term Plan are as follows:

The highlights

- Integrated teams in primary care, community health, social care
- A reduction in delayed discharges through various measures, including "same-day emergency care", development of urgent treatment centres (UTCs), stronger partnerships with local councils, and ring-fenced funding for primary care services, worth £4.5 billion/year by 2023/24
- New evidence-based NHS prevention programmes
- Funding allocations based on assessment of health inequalities and unmet need
- Allocation of funds to increase the number of planned operations and cut long waits
- A comprehensive NHS workforce implementation plan, underpinned by a new compact between frontline NHS leaders and national NSH leadership bodies, and an increase in undergraduate training programmes
- A plan to upgrade technology and digitally enabled care across the NHS, optimising personalised care, unlocking the potential of AI and linking clinical, genomic and other data, to support new medical breakthroughs
- Getting back onto a sustainable financial path, with savings of £700 million in reduced administrative costs and a revision to payment systems and incentives

Finance and productivity

- Commitments to return the provider sector to balance by 2020/21, and for all NHS organisations (commissioners and providers) to balance by 2023/24. To achieve this, NHS Improvement will deploy an accelerated turnaround process in the 30 financially worst-performing trusts, and a new financial recovery fund, initially £1.05 billion, will also be created for trusts in deficit who sign up to their control totals.
- Measures aimed at supporting delivery of integrated care and incentivising system-based working to improve population health. In 2019/20, as part of the process of moving towards system-control totals, sustainability and transformation partnerships (STPs) and integrated care systems (ICSs) will be given more flexibility to agree financially neutral changes, to control totals for individual organisations within their systems.

Workforce

- For nursing, the aim is to reduce the vacancy rate from 11.6 per cent to 5 per cent by 2028. To achieve this, as well as the previously announced 25 per cent increase in nurse undergraduate placements, the plan commits to funding a 25 per cent increase in clinical nursing placements from 2019/20, and an increase of up to 50 per cent from 2020/21.
- Commitment to increase medical school places from 6,000 to 7,500 per year, possibly more. There is also an ambition to shift the balance from specialised to generalist roles, in line with the needs of patients with multiple long-term conditions.
- The long-term ambition is to train more staff domestically. In the meantime, it emphasises the need for a continued inflow of international recruits.

Digital

- Digital technology underpins some of the plan's most ambitious patient-facing targets. The NHS app will act as a gateway for people to access services and information; by 2020/21, people will be able to use it to access their care plan and communications from health professionals.
- From 2024, patients will have a new "right" to access digital primary care services (e.g. online consultations), via either their existing practice or one of the emerging digital-first providers. By the end of the 10-year period covered by the plan, the vision is for people to be increasingly cared for and supported at home, using remote monitoring (via wearable devices) and digital tools.

Leadership and support of staff

- Range of actions to better support leaders, including doing more themselves to model the style of leadership they wish to see elsewhere in the system, and developing a new "NHS leadership code", which will enshrine expected cultural values and behaviours.
- Develop and embed cultures of compassion, inclusion and collaboration across the NHS. Specific actions include programmes and interventions to ensure a more diverse leadership cadre, a focus on increasing staff understanding of improvement knowledge and skills, and new pledges to better support senior leaders (including improving the approach to assurance and performance management).
- Do more to support current staff, including increasing investment in CPD, taking steps to promote flexibility and career development, and tackling bullying and harassment.

Role of patients and carers

- Fundamental shift required in the way that the NHS works alongside patients and individuals. Highlighting the need to create genuine partnerships between professionals and patients, the NHS commits to training staff to be able to have conversations that help people make the decisions that are right for them. There is also a commitment to increasing support for people to manage their own health, beginning in areas such as diabetes prevention and management.
- Focus on personalisation of care. Referrals to social prescribing schemes[34] will increase, broadening the range of support available, and the roll-out of personal health budgets will be accelerated, so that these are in place for up to 200,000 people by 2023/24.
- Stronger focus on supporting carers. This includes introducing quality markers for primary care, highlighting best practice in identifying carers, and providing them with appropriate support. It also encourages the national roll-out of carers' passports, which enable staff to identify someone as a carer and involve them in the patient's care, and promises a more proactive approach to supporting young carers.

Integrated care and population health

- Shift towards integrated care. A new accountability and performance framework will consolidate local performance measures, and a new integration index will measure patient and public views about local service integration.
- The move towards a more interconnected NHS will be supported by a "duty to collaborate" on providers and commissioners, while NHS England and NHS Improvement will continue efforts to streamline their functions.

Prevention and health inequalities

- Provision of alcohol-care teams in a quarter of hospitals with the highest rate of alcohol-dependence-related admissions, and a promise that by 2023/24, NHS-funded tobacco treatment services will be offered to all smokers admitted to hospital. There are also plans to introduce new programmes for specific diseases and conditions, and to scale up existing ones.
- A more concerted and systematic approach to reducing health inequalities', with a promise that action on inequalities will be central to everything that the NHS does. To support this ambition and to ensure that local plans and national programmes are focused on reducing inequalities, specific and measurable goals will be set.

---

[34] Social prescribing, sometimes referred to as community referral, is a means of enabling GPs, nurses and other primary care professionals to refer people to a range of local, non-clinical services.

Dental/oral health

Specifically related to dentistry and dental specialties, the NHS Long Term Plan pledges the following points:

- A plan to upgrade NHS support to all care home residents by 2023/24, with a pledge to support individuals in having good oral health
- The Starting Well Core initiative to support 24,000 dentists across England to see children from a young age and establish good oral health habits, to prevent the caries currently experienced by 25% of England's 5-year-old children.
- Ensuring that children with learning disabilities have their needs met by eyesight, hearing and dental services and are included in general screening services, as part of a pledge to ensure that all people with learning disability, autism, or both can live happier, healthier and longer lives.

13.4 Mid-Staffordshire NHS Foundation Trust: The two Francis inquiries

Background

In 2009 the Healthcare Commission (the old NHS regulator) published the findings of an investigation into failings in care at the Mid-Staffordshire NHS Foundation Trust. Focusing on problems at Stafford Hospital, the investigation found widespread failings in care. A local campaign group, Cure the NHS, led by Julie Bailey, whose mother died at the hospital, campaigned for an inquiry. The previous government ordered two Department of Health investigations, and then a secret inquiry led by Robert Francis QC, which lacked legal powers and focused on problems at the hospital, not wider failings.

The new coalition government ordered a full legal inquiry under Robert Francis QC, who was recognised to have led the first inquiry with sensitivity and care. This inquiry was charged with looking into failings by the various bodies and regulators that are supposed to prevent problems in care persisting.

One of the most worrying things about the scandal was that the trust had managed to achieve coveted "foundation status" whilst the problems were ongoing. This process required the support of the local Department of Health (known as Strategic Health Authorities); the NHS financial regulator, Monitor; and the Department of Health directly, including a government minister.

The Healthcare Commission report (March 2009)

The report highlighted a series of failures, particularly in A&E and AMU, and on some medical and surgical wards. Those concerns related to:

- Poor nursing standards
- Lack of effective management systems for emergencies
- Failure to identify and act on high mortality rates for patients admitted as emergencies
- A board detached from day-to-day reality of patient care
- Failure by the board to develop an open culture and to challenge current practice, despite information pointing to obvious problems

The report qualified the care received by patients as "appalling" and mentioned that this likely led to hundreds of unnecessary deaths. In March 2009, the Chairman was asked by Monitor to resign, and the chief executive of the trust resigned in order to avoid being suspended and investigated by the board.

In December 2009 a review published by the Royal College of Surgeons qualified the trust as "dysfunctional" and "frankly dangerous".

The first Francis inquiry (2010)

The first inquiry was designed to identify key failures and make recommendations. Led by Robert Francis QC, it identified a "bullying culture that was target focused in which the needs of the patients were ignored", and "an appalling failure at all levels".

Key failures identified included:

Board failures
- The board buried its head in the sand, failed to appreciate the enormity of the issues, reacted too slowly and generally downplayed the significance of many of the issues identified.
- The board responded to the healthcare commission report with denial. It showed no lack of urgency to resolve the issues raised.
- The CEO had concluded that high mortality rates were due to coding issues.
- The board set out to gain foundation status in order to improve the trust's governance, making it its number-one priority. This likely distracted it from dealing with more basic care-related issues.
- There was much focus on finances (the trust had been making losses for a few years). To save £10m (8% of its turnover), the trust set out to make cuts, including removing 150 posts. Wards were badly reorganised (separate floors for surgery and medicine, without carrying out any risk assessment), beds were cut and, consequently, patient care was compromised.
- Poor governance (clinical audit practice underdeveloped, critical incidents not reported or not acted upon, investigation of complaints done by staff from the area that caused the problem in the first place (and not seen by the board)).

Staff-related issues
- Too few consultants and nurses
- Constant change of management, leading to lack of leadership
- Doctors isolated from managers, the board and each other
- Some key individuals were unsafe
- Lack of attention to patient dignity (incontinent patients left in degrading conditions; patients left inadequately dressed in full public view; patients handled badly – sometimes by unskilled staff – causing pain and distress, rudeness, hostility; failure to refer to patients by name)
- Poor communication (lack of compassion and sensitivity, lack of information about patients' condition and care, lack of involvement of patients in decisions. Friends and family often ignored, failure to listen and reluctance to give

information, staff not communicating well with each other, wrong information provided to patients and relatives)
- Poor diagnosis and management (slow or premature discharge of patients, discharge from A&E without appropriate diagnosis or management, poor record keeping, poor or delayed diagnosis)
- Buzzers left unanswered

Cultural issues
- Patients concerned about insisting on proper care for fear of upsetting staff or of reprisals
- Staff distracted by their own mobile phones
- Staff not focused on basics (litter left on the floor, alcohol gel not replenished and therefore not used)
- Low staff morale

The second Francis inquiry (2013)

The second inquiry focused on commissioning, supervision and regulation of the hospital, querying particularly why such serious issues had not been identified earlier and acted upon sooner. The inquiry highlighted the following issues:

- Too much focus on finance, figures, targets and not enough on patient care (recent reforms emphasise outcomes rather than targets), and failure to put patients first
- Criticism of nursing training and lack of compassion in nursing profession
- Lack of accountability – attitude that "it's someone else's problem", e.g. managers vs. clinicians vs. board vs. politicians; key will be new Friends and Family test (at Mid Staffs only a quarter of staff would have recommended the hospital)
- Defensiveness, secrecy and complacency – focusing relentlessly on positives and closing eyes to negatives, i.e. poor standards
- Failure of doctors to speak up for patients
- Blind trust by PCTs and SHAs in the hospital's management and acceptance of hospital's reassurance without further checks.
- Insufficient levels of challenge by Monitor and CQC.
- Royal College of Nursing not supportive enough of its members when they raised concerns.
- Department of Health too remote.
- Concerns not raised by GPs until after the issues came to light.

Amongst the 290 recommendations the report made, here are some of the key ones:

- There should be more focus on compassion and caring in nursing recruitment, training and education.
- Patient safety should be the number-one priority, in both medical and nursing training and education.
- Individuals and organisations would have a duty to speak up (the government is in fact considering the possibility of criminal prosecution for staff who don't).
- Quality accounts should be published in a common format and made public.
- The profession of healthcare assistants should be regulated.
- For the elderly, one person should be in charge of individual patient care.
- The RCN should be either a royal college or a trade union.
- Patient involvement must be increased.
- Structural change is not the answer.

The government's response (27 March 2013)

- Duty of candour to be placed on NHS boards, to be honest about mistakes
- Consideration being given to making individual doctors and nurses criminally responsible for covering up errors
- New ratings system for hospitals and care homes, based on Ofsted scheme used in schools
- Posts of chief inspector of hospitals and care homes to be created, and possibly primary care
- Nurses to spend up to a year working as a healthcare assistant so they get experience providing basic care such as washing and dressing
- Managers who fail in their jobs to be barred from holding such positions in the future
- Code of conduct and minimum training standards for healthcare assistants, but not full registration scheme as recommended by inquiry
- Tough rules to be drawn up to allow trusts to be put into administration when basic standards are not met unless problems can be resolved quickly
- Department of Health civil servants to be forced to spend time on the front line of the NHS
- Prof. Don Berwick asked to set up an inquiry into "making harm a zero reality in the NHS" – National Advisory Panel on the Safety of Patients

13.5 Duty of candour

The new statutory duty of candour was introduced for NHS bodies in England (trusts, foundation trusts and special health authorities) on 27 November 2014, and applied to all other care providers registered with CQC from 1 April 2015. The obligations associated with the statutory duty of candour are contained in regulation 20 of The Health and Social Care Act 2008 (Regulated Activities) Regulations 2014. The key principles are:

1. Care organisations have a general duty to act in an open and transparent way in relation to care provided to patients. This means that an open and honest culture must exist throughout an organisation.

2. The statutory duty applies to organisations, not individuals, though it is clear from CQC guidance that it is expected that an organisation's staff cooperate with it to ensure the obligation is met.

3. As soon as is reasonably practicable after a notifiable patient safety incident occurs, the organisation must tell the patient (or their representative) about it in person.

4. The organisation has to give the patient a full explanation of what is known at the time, including what further inquiries will be carried out. Organisations must also provide an apology and keep a written record of the notification to the patient.

5. If the patient cannot be contacted or refuses to engage, a written record is to be kept of attempts to contact or to speak to him/her.

6. A notifiable patient-safety incident has a specific statutory meaning – any unintended or unexpected incident that occurred in respect of a service user during the provision of a regulated activity that, in the reasonable opinion of a healthcare professional, could result in, or appears to have resulted in:

   - The death of the service user, where the death relates directly to the incident rather than to the natural course of the service user's illness or underlying condition
   - Severe harm, moderate harm, or prolonged psychological harm to the service user

"Severe harm" means a permanent lessening of bodily, sensory, motor, physiologic or intellectual functions, including removal of the wrong limb or organ or brain damage, which is related directly to the incident and not related to the natural course of the service user's illness or underlying condition.

"Moderate harm" means harm that requires a moderate increase in treatment (that is, an unplanned return to surgery, an unplanned re-admission, a prolonged episode of care, extra time in hospital or as an outpatient, cancelling of treatment, or transfer to another treatment area (such as intensive care); and significant, but not permanent, harm.

7. There is a statutory duty to provide reasonable support to the patient. Reasonable support could be providing an interpreter to ensure discussions are understood, or giving emotional support to the patient following a notifiable patient safety incident.

Once the patient has been told in person about the notifiable patient-safety incident, the organisation must provide the patient with a written note of the discussion, and copies of correspondence must be kept.

It is worth knowing defined "never events" in dentistry. These take their cue from surgical never events:

- Wrong site surgery, including wrong tooth extraction (but not extraction of incorrect deciduous teeth, unless performed under general anaesthesia)
- Wrong site surgery includes wrong site blocks for pain relief, but a wrong side interior alveolar nerve block will no longer be regarded as a never event
- Wrong implants/prosthesis
- Retained foreign objects post-procedure

A comprehensive suggestion of dental-specific never events can be found in the eDelphi survey.[35]

The General Dental Council (GDC) has published specific guidance on the professional duty of candour[36]. Before treatment starts, it is important that patients understand their options and the benefits and risks of those options. Patients should be empowered to make an informed decision. When things go wrong, registrants must:

---

[35] Ensaldo-Carrasco E, et al. Developing agreement on never events in primary care dentistry: an international eDelphi study. *Br Dent J* 2018;224:733–740.
[36] https://www.gdc-uk.org/docs/default-source/the-professional-duty-of-candour/duty-of-candour.pdf?sfvrsn=cba6dd3e_4

1. Tell the patient
2. Apologise

    a.   Explain what happened
    b.   Explain what has been done to put matters right
    c.   Describe what will be done to stop the same thing happening to someone else (if relevant)

3. Offer an appropriate remedy or support to put matters right
4. Explain the short- and long-term effects

13.6 Maintaining registration and CPD

The rules surrounding continuing professional development (CPD) changed recently, with the introduction of the Enhanced CPD Scheme by the GDC in 2018, applicable to all dental care professionals (DCPs). The key consideration is that there is not a "one size fits all" approach, but CPD should be tailored to the individual roles, work and patient cohort of different clinicians.

Dentists have to do a minimum of 100 hours in every five-year cycle for CPD, with at least 10 hours done every two years. The CPD record maintained by a registrant needs to include a personal development plan (PDP), a log of CPD activity and documentary evidence for all activity, as well as an element of reflection. This is distinct from the previous rules regarding CPD that differentiated "verifiable" CPD from non-verifiable CPD, which is no longer the case. Essentially, whilst the GDC encourages continued CPD outside of the formal requirement, only verifiable CPD now needs to be declared on an annual basis.

Each CPD activity must have at least one of the GDC development outcomes:

A. Effective communication with patients, the dental team and others across dentistry, including when obtaining consent, dealing with complaints and raising concerns when patients are at risk

B. Effective management of self and effective management of others or effective work with others in the dental team, in the interests of patients; providing constructive leadership where appropriate

C. Maintenance and development of knowledge and skill within your field of practice

D. Maintenance of skills, behaviours and attitudes which maintain patient confidence in you and the dental profession and put patients' interests first[37]

The GDC recommends a wide breadth of activity contribute towards CPD requirements including (but not limited to): e-learning, courses, lectures, hand-on training or workshops, clinical audit and conferences. There are however criteria for verifiable CPD that are more stringent than in the past with providers being subject to guidance laid out in the GDC document *Enhanced CPD guidance for providers*.[38]

---

[37] General Dental Council document *Enhanced CPD guidance:* https://www.gdc-uk.org/docs/default-source/enhanced-cpd-scheme-2018/enhanced-cpd-guidance-for-professionals.pdf?sfvrsn=edbe677f_4)
[38] https://www.gdc-uk.org/docs/default-source/enhanced-cpd-scheme-2018/cpd-provider-guidance.pdf?sfvrsn=63766c6a_2

All delegates/participants should receive certification that should state:

- Subject/learning content
- GDC development outcomes from the list above
- Date(s) undertaken
- Total number of hours
- The name of the delegate/participant
- That there is a quality assurance (QA) process in place, with a named individual/organisation responsible
- Confirmation that the information given is full and accurate

Continued registration with the GDC is contingent on keeping up with CPD requirements, meeting the annual retention fee (ARF) and ensuring that indemnity arrangements are in place appropriate to a registrant's sphere of practice. Remember that GDC registration is not just for dentists and also encompasses dental nurses, dental technicians, dental therapists, dental hygienists, orthodontic therapists and clinical dental technicians, all classed as dental care professionals (DCPs). Dentists may also be temporary registrants (TRs) (e.g. overseas-qualified and undertaking approved training programmes in the United Kingdom) or visiting dental practitioners (VPs), under EU directive 2004/38/EC, which is still current at the time of writing.

13.7 The NHS in Wales, Scotland and Northern Ireland

There are virtually no questions being asked on political issues in interviews in Wales, Scotland and Northern Ireland. We have set out below basic information, which will give an indication of the key features of the health system in each country.

Wales

The reorganisation of NHS Wales, which came into effect on 1 October 2009, created single local health organisations that are responsible for delivering all healthcare services within a geographical area, rather than the trust and local health board system that existed previously. The reorganisation abolished the internal market.

There are seven health boards. In Wales, healthcare funding is still based on block contracts between Welsh commissioners and the relevant providers. Funding to hospitals from Welsh commissioners is therefore based on historical activity and funding levels, as a guide for the expected number of treatments over the coming year. Clinical activities are not funded on the basis of actual activities provided. Instead, an overall figure of anticipated activity is agreed in advance between the commissioner and the provider.

The Health and Social Services budget is £6 billion – 40% of the Welsh Assembly's total budget. On 1 April 2007, the NHS prescription charge was abolished for people in Wales.

Dentistry in Wales follows the Units of Dental Activity (UDA) system, as followed in England. Again, the National Assembly's Health, Social Care and Sport Committee has echoed sentiments from reviews in England, with concerns regarding dentists being discouraged from taking on high-needs patients with the current system of remuneration. As such, there have been calls for a more flexible system and a shift of focus onto prevention and quality of care.

Scotland

The Scottish Government Health Directorate (SGHD) has responsibility for NHS Scotland as well as the development and implementation of community health policy. The SGHD undertakes the central management of NHS Scotland and heads a management executive, which oversees the activity of the 14 regional NHS boards.

The roles of the health boards include strategic leadership and performance management of the entire local NHS system in their areas, and assurance that services are delivered safely, effectively and cost-efficiently. The 14 NHS boards are ultimately responsible for the commissioning, provision and management of the full range of health services, in an area including hospitals and general practice.

Payment to hospitals is on a block-contract basis. Like Wales, Scotland offers free prescriptions to its residents. The budget for NHS Scotland is £11 billion, just over one third of the Scottish government's annual budget.

Dentistry in Northern Ireland and Scotland moved in a different direction from that in England, with the introduction of the 2006 contract, with both Northern Ireland and Scotland keeping an existing statement of dental remuneration and FFS payment system, rather than the retrospective UDA system.

Northern Ireland

In Northern Ireland the National Health Service is referred to as "HSC", or "Health and Social Care". Just like the other NHS, it is free at the point of delivery, but it also provides social care services such as home care services, family and children's services, day-care services and social work services.

The Department of Health, Social Services and Public Safety has overall authority for health and social care services. Services are commissioned by the health and social care board and provided by five health and social care trusts – Belfast, the largest of the five, South Eastern, Southern, Northern and Western.

The health and social care board sits between the department and trusts, and is responsible for commissioning services, managing resources and performance improvement. Inside the board there are local commissioning groups (LCGs), focusing on the planning and resourcing of services. The LCGs cover the same geographical areas as the five health and social care trusts.

The budget for the Department of Health, Social Services and Public Safety is £4 billion: 40% of the Northern Ireland Executive's annual budget.

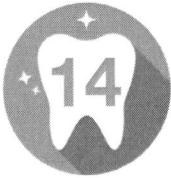

14 Body language and dress code

Much has been written about body language, and you may find various statistics quoted, such as body language representing about 60% of your communication.

Whilst there is no doubt that body language is important in helping you make a good impression, one should not forget that, ultimately, your body language is a reflection of your confidence and that confidence is not something that you acquire solely by smiling politely and moving your arms properly. There is a danger that a candidate may concentrate heavily on his/her appearance, at the expense of building content and structure into his/her answers.

As you gain more and more confidence through your preparation, your body language will change and will open up naturally. We would therefore recommend that you do not worry about it until you are well advanced in your preparation.

The key rules of body language

If your interview consists of several stations of 10 minutes each, you will need to build a rapport and make a good impression quickly. Here are a few key rules that you will need to follow:

- **Eye contact**
  This is the most crucial part of your relationship with the interviewers, as far as body language is concerned. No one will be interested in listening to someone who is not looking straight at them, so make sure that you maintain good eye contact with whoever is asking you the question. Occasionally, look at the other person too, so that they feel included.

- **Seat position**
  If you are sitting behind a table, make sure that you are not too close or too far from the table. If you are too close, you will have difficulty relaxing, and your elbows will also be forced to rest on the table. The interviewers would feel that you are invading their space and may be forced to back away from you. If you are too far from the table, you will either start slouching in your seat, giving the impression that you don't really care, or you will lean forward, reaching for the table. Not only will you get lower back pains, but you will also appear very casual.

A good distance is about 10cm from the table so that your arms can rest on the table comfortably, with your elbows remaining outside the table and not on it.

- **Arm positions**
  Many candidates find it comfortable to have their hands under the table. This gives an impression of timidity and of trying to hide behind the furniture. You need to project an image of quiet confidence, and having your hands on the table will help you achieve that.

- **Hand movements**
  It is perfectly acceptable to move your hands if it is part of your personality. Don't force yourself if it doesn't come naturally to you, though. If you are someone whose hands tend to move naturally, make sure that you contain that movement to the space in front of you and no higher than chest level; otherwise your hand movements will start obstructing your face.

Dress code

There are hundreds of ways in which you can make a good impression with your dress code and, in a way, it would be patronising to impose a general way of dressing. What matters is that you are comfortable in your clothes and that they are fit for the purpose of a professional meeting. It often helps to mirror the dress code of those interviewing you (generally conservative). There are some general rules that will make a difference in the way in which people perceive you, though:

- **Dress to frame your face**
  The focal point should be your face; therefore, you want to frame your face by wearing darker colours on the outside and lighter colours on the inside. For men, this will mean a shirt of light tone and for women a light-coloured blouse. This should be complemented by a dark-toned suit.

- **Look neat**
  If you wear a beard, make sure you trim it. If you wear make-up, don't overdo it. Clip your nails, tidy your hair, and make sure none of it obstructs your face. We know it sounds obvious, but you would be surprised.

- **Avoid distracting features**
  Continuing on the theme of your face being the focal point, avoid any features or accessories that may draw the eye to the wrong places. In particular, no sequins (they make wonderful disco balls when light reflects off them), no brooches, no ribbons, poppies, or other symbols that are either too big or too bright in colour. Small items of jewellery may be okay, providing they do not steal the limelight away from you and do not draw the attention away from your face.

PRACTICAL INTERVIEW STATIONS

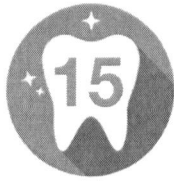

15 Communication station

Communication/role-play stations have become increasingly common at interviews in many specialties. They are based on realistic scenarios, with the patient being played either by an interviewer or a professional actor. Role plays are designed to test your communication skills more than your clinical skills – though, inevitably, a relevant clinical knowledge is essential to perform well – and the marking schemes reflect this, i.e. if you have excellent communication skills but talk rubbish, you will not pass the station.

Such stations are commonly a feature of dental specialty recruitment and were included in 2019 for both pre- and post-CCST interviews for paediatric dentistry (entry points at ST1 and ST4, respectively), oral surgery and orthodontics, as examples.

The marking scheme

A variety of marking schemes has been used in the past for communication/role-play stations. Typically, two interviewers would assess the candidate on a range of communication criteria.

As stated above, in role-play scenarios and communication stations, candidates are commonly marked on aspects set apart from technical knowledge and detail that may contribute relatively little to the overall mark. More commonly, other aspects are examined and marked, such as:

- Listening abilities
- Verbal communication, e.g. clarity of explanation
- Non-verbal communication
- Developing a rapport
- Overall impression

The role player may be asked to contribute a mark in some instances, but may also be asked on their opinion of how they felt about a particular candidate, was the explanation clear, their manner reassuring, etc.

Criteria will vary in their wording and in the manner in which they are grouped, but generally speaking, the expectations and overall criteria are the same. A good example of this is available online for orthodontics.[39] Scores are given against anchor statements, with the following being examples:

- **Score 0:** "Use expressions or words that would not be understood by the listener throughout the interview"
- **Score 1:** "Frequently use expressions or words that would not be understood by the listener"
- **Score 2:** "Occasionally use expressions or words that would not be understood by the listener"
- **Score 3:** "Seldom use expressions or words that would not be understood by the listener"
- **Score 4:** "Never use expressions or words that would not be understood by the listener"

Timing and preparation time

Timing will vary between specialties, but as a guide, one could look at the description for the 2019 interview for paediatric dentistry:

- Pre-CCST: Applicants observed by two clinicians and assessed on interaction with a "parent" by the clinicians and the role player, with 10 minutes' preparation time before entering the station, consisting of a review of "a scenario"
- Post-CCST: Applicants observed by two clinicians and assessed on interaction by clinicians and role player, but with 20 minutes' preparation time, encompassing a review of "related clinical documents"

Make sure you make the best use of that preparation time to read the brief given to you and the patient's history so that:

- You do not miss any crucial information during the consultation

- You do not waste time during the consultation asking the patient about information that you have been told you already know; some actors may have been instructed to act angry if they have to repeat information that is in the brief

---

[39]https://madeinheene.hee.nhs.uk/Portals/13/Clinical%20Communication%20Station%2020 19%20-%20Descriptors.pdf

Running the role play

In order to score well, you will need to ensure that you address the following:

Understanding of the impact of the environment on the consultation
In some role plays, the room will be set up with the dentist's and the patient's chairs in positions that may not be ideal to build a rapport with the patient/parent. If you feel it appropriate, you may want to move your chair and the patient's chair so that they are at an appropriate distance. If there is a table, you should ensure that you are not sitting across the table from the patient but that you are separated only by a corner of the table.

Introduction
Greet the patient by name if the brief gives it to you. Introduce yourself by name. Shake their hand if the patient is willing to accept, and take the patient to the seat reserved for them (some actors may be instructed to remain standing until you invite them to sit down. If the situation warrants it, ask if they have come accompanied and if they want their relative or friend to sit in on the conversation. If you have been given a task (e.g. explaining a near miss or untoward event), then start by giving an overview of how and for how long the conversation will run, and say that you will end with a clear, agreed management plan. If you or the department has caused the patient some harm, it is important to start with an apology.

Encourage the patient to tell you about the problem, using open questions such as "What can I do for you today?" If the patient has been recalled to see you for a specific purpose, you can start more directly, by explaining the reason for the recall.

Listening and empathy
When discussing the issue at stake with the patient, allow the patient time to talk. Do not interrupt them unless you feel that you really need to. There are times when one needs to learn to keep quiet.

Be attentive to what they are telling you. The actor will have been primed to drop certain clues into the conversation, either voluntarily or taking one of your questions as a cue. In role play, candidates are often so obsessed with what they should do next that they sometimes forget to listen to the patient.

Throughout the conversation, observe the patient's behaviour. Listening does not necessarily mean only hearing their words. You can pick up a lot of information by observing their body language. An awkward body language may give you clues about something that the patient is not telling you or is feeling embarrassed or scared about.

If the patient is silent or uncommunicative, encourage them by asking open questions. If the patient is distressed, it may also prove valuable to simply allow the situation to remain silent for a while, if talking does not help. This may help them regain their composure.

History taking, diagnosis and clinical information
Ask all questions relevant to the scenario and explain any necessary points. Try not to ask for information that you should already know from the brief, as you may irritate the patient. However, if you feel the need to confirm some information with the patient, either because the brief is ambiguous or the patient has contradicted information that you were given, then you may double-check.

Explain your diagnosis and/or treatment plan to the patient. Use words that are appropriate for the patient. Ensure that the patient understands what you are explaining; if necessary, ask them to confirm their understanding by repeating in their own words what they have understood and by using questions such as "Is there anything that you do not understand?" or "Is there anything that you would like me to clarify?" If appropriate, explain using different methods or media (some spare paper may be made available to you).

Do not go into overdrive on the clinical section of your consultation at the expense of everything else. You would be surprised at how little this accounts for in the overall marking scheme on these stations. Remember that the premise is that clinical knowledge and skills can be taught to you on the training programme, but good interpersonal skills are harder to teach and therefore need to be established ideally at the outset.

Holistic and psychosocial needs
The interviewers will be testing your ability to identify the various needs of the patient and how you address them during the consultation. Consider the physical aspects of the problem, but also the psychological and social sides. How is the patient coping? What is the impact on their self-image and self-confidence? What social constraints are there in seeking treatment (e.g. travel, family responsibilities, financial issues)? Make sure that you elicit the patient's ideas, concerns and expectations, as the textbook "right" answer for the condition is not necessarily the right answer for the patient concerned!

Body language
The manner in which you attempt to build a rapport with the patient, and the appropriateness of your body language, play an important role in your success at handling any role play. Make sure that you keep an open posture (no crossed arms), avoid being above or too close to them, lean slightly forward to show empathy when required, nod in the right places and, most important of all, maintain good eye contact with the patient to maintain that crucial rapport. Eye contact will also enable you to

read the patient's emotions and possible discomfort, which could provide valuable clues. If they look like they may cry, a hand on their hand or shoulder may be appropriate, or you could pass them some tissues.

The unexpected

Some role plays are fairly mainstream (i.e. they attempt to replicate a normal consultation or scenario, without any particular surprises). Others have twists and turns, which may catch you off guard. This may include a patient who suddenly becomes irate; a patient who suddenly withdraws, refuses to say any more and looks down; a patient who cannot speak a word of English; or a patient who takes you onto a completely unexpected path.

When this happens, you must always remember that it is a game, i.e. that this was planned. Rather than give up, try to remain calm and see how you can help the situation along. If the patient has walked out, see if you can get them back by using a more diplomatic approach. If the patient is not talking, don't just look at the examiners in despair; see if you can re-engage. If the patient throws you off guard by mentioning issues that you were not expecting, don't look flustered or stunned. If you are, then ask the patient to elaborate on what they have just said; it will give you some time to regain your composure (and might help you score some listening points). If a patient is angry, slow down the speed of your conversation and become quieter; hopefully they will match you.

Ending the consultation

Role plays can be conducted in different manners. In some cases, the interviewers will let you know when you have two minutes left, but in many cases they won't. The first you will hear from them is the sound of a bell and a "Thank you – you can move to the next station" grunt. Make sure that you keep track of time so that, if possible, you can draw the conversation to a natural close. Most marking schemes will include an allowance for your conclusion or summary, so make sure you get there. If you feel that you are likely to run out of time because you went off on a tangent or allowed the patient a bit too much space, then make a quick assessment of the situation and determine whether it is worth sacrificing one mark for not having a conclusion but gaining several more marks by addressing several other important issues instead.

Towards the end of the consultation, you should summarise to the patient what action is being proposed and what they have agreed to. You should also explain whether follow-up will be required and when. Thank them for coming and escort them to the door.

Ask yourself whether you have forgotten any important aspects, and cover these as necessary. If not, then don't be afraid of terminating the exercise a few minutes early. It is better to end on a confident note than to waffle on for two minutes to kill time.

Examples of role plays

Topics will obviously vary per specialty, but here are some theoretical examples.

- Explaining to a parent the finding of a compound odontome, the nature of the diagnosis and the possible treatment plan

- Consenting a patient for fixed appliance therapy, and discussing the need for extraction of healthy teeth and possible risks, e.g. root resorption

- Handling a never event with a patient, of a wrong tooth extraction carried out by a DCT, on the clinic where you were the assigned middle grade clinician

- Explaining an unforeseen complication under day case general anaesthesia, e.g. displaced root of a lower third molar into the sublingual space

- Relaying to a patient a lost biopsy specimen for a suspected benign lesion

- Discussing a diagnosis of hypodontia, and a treatment plan, and/or interfacing with the multidisciplinary team

- A new diagnosis of oral epithelial dysplasia and need for ongoing review in a patient who is the main carer for his partner who has Alzheimer's

- Dealing with a tearful mum of a patient requiring multiple extractions for fixed appliance therapy

- Dealing with a patient, who developed a dry socket following a wisdom tooth extraction, who insists that they should have been given antibiotics post-operatively

The list is far from exhaustive but you get the idea! There may be hidden agendas, social circumstances, accusations of incompetence of your colleagues and a fair amount of ire! Remember to stay calm, actively listen and take it all in your stride!

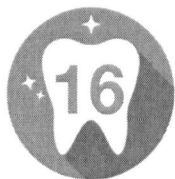

16 Presentation station

Presentations are a recruitment tool that is on the increase. They have been a common feature at consultant interviews for some time and may yet find their way into DCT and ST recruitment, although for the time being do not seem to have made an appearance!

What is being assessed?

Through your presentation, the interviewers will be assessing:

- Your general presentation skills (confidence, ability to engage an audience, etc)

- Your ability to communicate your ideas clearly, concisely, using an approach suited to the topic and the audience; this will include marks for the clarity of the slides and their relevance

- The content of the presentation, i.e. the appropriateness and maturity of the content

- Your time management and organisational skills, i.e. your ability to stick to time, to allocate appropriate timing to each of the sections in your talk, etc

Similar to the communication/role-play station, the marking scheme is likely to score each of the above out of four, the combined marks of the two assessors forming the candidate's final score.

Preparation time and duration

Presentations generally vary in length between 5 and 10 minutes. Whilst in some specialties you may be asked to prepare a presentation in advance (the details being communicated to you in the invitation letter), in others you are likely to be placed on the spot, with the presentation topic being given to you just 45 minutes before you are due to present. Slides or overheads are usually allowed, though some restrict their number, whilst others require you to speak without visual aids. It is important to clarify the equipment that will be available on the day and then have several failsafe backup options. We have all seen people fail to get their projector working, even at national meetings. Ways to bring digital media include: CD, memory stick, uploaded to the web or emailed to the department. It may be worth copying onto transparencies for an overhead projector or bringing handouts.

Example of topics

Presentation topics are very varied. They generally fall under three different categories:

Generic
- Tell us about yourself.
- What can you contribute to this specialty?
- How do you see your career developing, what skills do you have and which would you wish to gain?
- Why do you think you will make a good <xxx>?

Political
- How do current NHS changes impact on this specialty?
- How can this specialty become more efficient?
- How will you make sure that you become a good consultant when working hours are being decreased?

Personal
- Tell us about your hobbies.
- How have your strengths and weaknesses informed your career choice?

Occasionally, you may be asked to talk about some non-work-related topic of your choice. This has led to candidates making presentations on topics as varied as:
- How to teach cricket to 10-year-old children
- How to fly a helicopter
- The history of chocolate
- Silver hallmarking

Essentially, presentations can be regarded as extended interview questions, which you have 10 minutes rather than 2 minutes to answer. In that sense, similar principles apply with regard to the need to structure the information around three or four themes or ideas, and the need to make the information memorable by giving examples. There is nothing worse than a presentation which is too theoretical. Relate it to your audience.

Key principles

There are a few rules that you will need to remember during your preparation.

Keep the number of slides to a minimum
The rule of thumb is to have no more than one slide per 90 seconds of talk. Therefore, a 10-minute presentation should contain no more than six or seven slides. If your talk

is organised around four central ideas (as it should be), then you would need only one slide for each, plus an introduction and a summary slide, making six slides in total.

Keep the slides short and simple – the 4 by 4 rule

Never forget that the slides are there to support your presentation and help your audience. They are not there to replace your notes because you can't be bothered to learn your talk. If the slides are too busy, then the interviewers will struggle to read them and to listen to you at the same time. The best slides are those that stick to the main principles and allow the audience to focus their attention on the candidate. As a general rule, you should have no more than 4 bullet points, each with no more than 4 words (this is called the "4 by 4 rule").

You should also ensure that any text written on the slides is large enough to be seen from a distance. You may want to ask beforehand whether the slides will be projected onto a screen (even if through an overhead projector) or simply read from a laptop. Whatever method they choose, your slides should be readable from a laptop screen that is three metres away. If they are not, then there is either too much text or the font size is too small. Generally, have high contrast between text and background (e.g. black on white or white/yellow on dark blue).

Vary your slides and make them accessible

Always think whether there is a more interesting way of representing your message than through standard bullet points. For example, if you want to convey that there are four issues that the NHS is focusing on currently, you could simply list them as bullet points, for example:

- Efficiency
- Training
- Quality
- Profitability

Alternatively, I could convey the same with four pictures on your slide:

- Efficiency: a picture of an organised or a chaotic unit
- Training: a picture of a ward round, or of a lecture
- Quality: a picture of a "tick"
- Profitability: a picture of a money bag or a pound sign

Pictures, graphics and other means of visual representation are often very powerful and, in the meantime, your audience does not spend hours trying to decipher whole lines of text, written in font size 8, in a desperate bid to make it all fit onto the page. Some of the best presentations we have seen included one candidate who used pictures only, no words, and a candidate who simply opted to use no visual aids. The effect it had was that the interviewers could then pay full attention to his talk. It is worth checking whether slides are essential (i.e. whether their quality will be judged) or whether they are just accepted, as this may give you ideas for how to make your talk more interesting. Try to avoid being too flashy or using complicated animations, transitions and movies, even if you are an expert. The interviewers are likely to use an old version of Windows, an old version of Microsoft Office and a slow computer.

Prepare a good speech, rehearse and take your time to deliver it
At the risk of stating the obvious, you must make sure that you rehearse your presentation many times so that you know it well, even without any visual aids. You should rehearse the presentation at least four times, two of which should be under time pressure, ideally in front of a scary panel!

Your speech, and not the slides, should be the main focus of the presentation. If you have prepared your visual aids properly, there should still be plenty of information that you need to add verbally to your presentation. Your speech will bring colour to your presentation, will bring personal reflection onto your ideas, and will guide the audience through their journey of discovery.

As a rule, you should allow approximately 160 words per minute of speech. If you have to speak too quickly to get to the end of the presentation within the allocated time, then you have too much information. Go back to the drawing board and see if all the information that you are presenting is relevant. If it isn't relevant, or if it confuses matters, then take it out. Be ruthless: the simpler the presentation, the better. Often the problem is linked to a lack of proper structure or the wrong structure. See if you can reorganise the information using different headings. Having more complex slides also increases the risk of you being out of synch with them, and that is confusing for the audience.

Prepare some notes
During the presentation itself, it is preferable that you do not use notes. The danger of using notes is that you will inevitably be tempted to look at them. Also, reading them will make you sound wooden. However, you should bring a set with you, just in case you have a memory gap. Make sure that they are hidden from you in your jacket pocket and that they are in a suitably small size (i.e. postcard size rather than A4) so that you can just pull them out of your pocket if need be without looking too flustered.

Watch your voice and delivery
- Your voice must be confident and normally loud.
- Avoid dropping your voice at the end of your sentences.
- Pause briefly between each slide. You might know your topic well, but your audience will need time to keep up with you.
- Find good ways to link the slides.
- Do not rush your delivery.

Watch your body language

- Smile! Even a nervous smile is more endearing than a depressed or terrorised look.
- Adopt a natural stance. This means having your feet 25cm apart, with your knees very slightly bent. Relax your shoulders.
- Be aware of your natural habits. Some people have a tendency to play with loose change in their pockets, to sway from one foot to the other, to play with a pen or their watchstrap. You must be able to identify those habits and squash them before someone on the panel finds them irritating.
- Keep your hands in front of your belly. You can move them but not in an exaggerated fashion.

How to prepare

A common problem with presentations is the lack of clarity and simplicity in the message that the candidates want to convey. This results in complicated and confused slides, which then translates into a poor delivery. To perform well, you will first need to make sure that you have your story in the right order. Once you have looked at the topic, start talking about it in your head or aloud and see what comes out. Once you have perfected the story, you will be much better able to identify the key points that form its structure and its logic. Those points will form the backbone of your presentation and will dictate your slides. If you commit your thoughts too early to paper or to slides, you will lose flexibility. You will be reluctant to change the order of your slides or review the entire structure of your talk, for fear of having wasted your preparation time. Not committing your talk to paper too early will enable you to adopt a totally different approach, without having to rewrite a lot of material. Try to reframe from another's point of view. Try taking a system (helicopter) view, or see the topic from the point of view of a commissioner or a patient or the panel themselves. What would be important or interesting for each of these stakeholders?

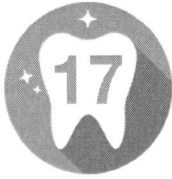

Group discussion station

Group discussions are yet to make an appearance, but are worth including as a possible interview format, which may be introduced and have been used elsewhere.

Format of the group discussion

Group discussions typically last 20 minutes. There will usually be four people in each group, sitting around a table, with each being assessed by an external observer. In some cases, there may be just one observer for two candidates. The team is given a brief shortly before the session commences and, at the agreed time, the required discussion needs to start.

There are two main types of group discussions:

- **Normal discussion**
  The group is given a general topic of discussion and has to debate the issues involved. In many cases, the discussion is based on a simple two-line brief such as an ethical issue. In other cases, the information provided is more comprehensive and may include, for example, a letter of complaint addressed to your consultant, or extracts from patient notes. In other, more complex group discussions, the candidates may actually be given different pieces of information; for example, one candidate may have a summary of the notes, another candidate will be given a complaint letter, and another an abstract from a report.

- **Role-play group discussion**
  In this type of group discussion, each candidate is allocated a different role. One candidate may be playing the DCT, another candidate a dental care professional, another candidate the consultant from one specialty and the fourth candidate a consultant from an interfacing specialty. The roles obviously depend on the type of scenario given.

What the assessors are looking for

Much as it is tempting to show off your knowledge of the topic being discussed, this is only one of the areas that the assessors will be looking for. Indeed, if they wanted to test your knowledge, they would either ask you a direct question in a normal interview setting or ask you to do a presentation.

The assessors will, however, be far more interested in the manner in which you interact with the rest of the group. This can be very complex, to assess when people can have such diverse personalities. Some candidates will be natural leaders and they may well feel at ease driving the conversation. Other candidates may be good facilitators, i.e. they get on well with most people and are able to keep the peace. Others still may contribute much to the team by generating content and ideas but could not lead or facilitate.

What the interviewers will be looking at, therefore, is a general pattern of behaviour that fits well within a team, and your interaction with others, whatever your personality. This will include:

- Your general contribution to the discussion (which can include active listening, support of others and encouraging opinions from the quieter members)

- Your problem-solving abilities

- Your general interaction with others, including your body language and the appropriateness of your behaviour (e.g. empathy, sensitivity, situation awareness)

- Your ability to cope with the challenges of working within a team (e.g. pushy colleagues, uncooperative people, quiet people)

- Clarity of communication and assertiveness if necessary

- Your ability to influence/negotiate with people, i.e. to rally people to your point of view without making them feel coerced

Dealing with difficulties within the group

Going round in circles
There may be a time when the conversation has ceased to be productive and the team has either gone off on a tangent or is caught in a vicious circle. In such cases, you would score marks for enabling the team to get back on track by gently reminding everyone of the original goal and pointing out in a non-threatening manner that you all got lost. Bring the focus back to the patient, to avoid making things confrontational.

Awkward silences

The team may have reached a natural break in the discussion, or it may be that no one dares speak in case they say something stupid. If this happens, you should encourage the team to summarise the discussion so far, to set out the main themes that could be discussed and then to ensure that the points are dealt with systematically. If the conversation has ended because all points were discussed, then finish the exercise early; do not go on waffling until the bell rings.

Overbearing colleagues

Some talk a lot because they are extroverts; extroverts tend to think while they talk and may actually change their opinion by 180 degrees very quickly. Others may talk a lot due to nerves. There will always been one in the group who will have misunderstood the point of the exercise, thinking that he will look clever by showing off his knowledge of the topic being discussed.

Such people can do themselves much damage but can also take you down with them if you are not careful. Indeed, by occupying the space and monopolising the time available, they do not allow you the platform that you need to show off your own team-playing skills.

If you are that person, then make sure you allow others to have a say and encourage them. If you are faced with such a colleague, the best way to handle the situation with different strategies is:

- Asking others what they feel about what this person has said

- Asking for a break in the discussions so that you can summarise the points made so far

- Directly letting the colleague know that it would be useful for others to comment so that you can get different perspectives on the problem

Silent colleague

Some are silent because they are introverts, doing lots of thinking in their heads and then waiting to give a considered answer. Ask them directly, and wait for seven to eight seconds for a reply. Others may just feel uncomfortable with the role-play technique, be anxious as it is part of the interview, or just not know the answer.

By themselves, silent colleagues may not feel like a threat because they give you the floor. But in fact, if you ignore them and do not encourage them, you may be marked down. Pay attention to those around so that you can spot them.

If you are that person, then you will need to make an effort to participate, at least by encouraging others. No silent candidate will score anything. If you want to demonstrate that you are a good listener, then you will need to make sure that you demonstrate this, not just by listening but also by summarising the points made so far and helping the team move forward.

If you are faced with a silent colleague, try to encourage them to participate by asking for their opinion at an appropriate moment. If they refuse to be involved, then do not force them, as it would count against you, but demonstrate at least that you are making an effort.

USEFUL
RESOURCES

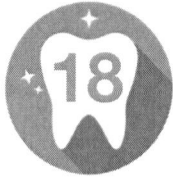

18 Action and power words

The vocabulary and turns of phrase that you use at an interview will make a big difference to the way in which your answers are perceived by the interviewers, and to the confidence and maturity that you exude.

Part of your maturity and confidence will come from the spontaneity and fluency of your answers, both of which can be addressed through practice, but much of which will come from using words that convey your meaning powerfully.

The impact of action and power words

Consider these sentences:
- I would be happy to play a role in teaching.
- I have been lucky to be involved in audit over the past two years.
- I have had the opportunity to be involved in research.
- My consultant has asked me to be involved in research.
- I have been part of a team that developed guidelines on <xxx>.

None of these really convey a strong sense of commitment and enthusiasm. At an interview, saying such sentences would be okay in small doses, but if repeated too often, they will give the feeling that you are not in control of your career and that you are adopting a passive stance.

- "I would be happy" basically means "Ask me nicely and I would do it".
- "I have been lucky" conveys that you did not choose to get involved but that you rely on others to give you opportunities.
- "I have had the opportunity" makes you rely on the chance that someone (or fate) will create an opportunity where you can get involved.
- "My consultant has asked me" may be what actually happened, but again, it makes you look dependent and not in charge of your destiny.
- "I have been part of a team" may be okay as an introduction if you then go on to talk about yourself, but does not convey your own role and, as such, runs the risk that you may be selling the achievement of the team rather than your own.

There are tighter, more assertive and more powerful ways of selling yourself, by using what is termed "power" or "action" words. For example:
- "I have <u>developed a strong interest</u> in teaching and am very <u>keen to take on</u> a more prominent role over the next few years."

- "I have <u>played a key role</u> in managing audit projects, from data collection to presentation stage."
- "I <u>discussed with my consultant</u> a number of research opportunities, following which I <u>embarked on a project</u> that looked at <xxx>"
- "I <u>reviewed</u> our morbidity rate following procedure <xxx> and, as a result, I <u>worked closely</u> with two of my colleagues to introduce new guidelines on <yyy>."

These power words will help you convey your meaning in a more distinct manner and will make a lot of difference to your final mark.

List of action and power words

Here is a list of over 500 power words, which you can use to increase the strength of your answers. These can be used not only in formal interview questions, but also in role play and group discussions.

Abbreviated	Abolished	Abridged	Absolved
Absorbed	Accelerated	Acclimated	Accompanied
Achieved	Acquired	Acted	Activated
Actuated	Adapted	Added	Addressed
Adhered	Adjusted	Administered	Admitted
Adopted	Advanced	Advertised	Advised
Advocated	Affected	Aided	Aired
Allocated	Altered	Amended	Amplified
Analysed	Answered	Anticipated	Applied
Appointed	Appraised	Approached	Approved
Arbitrated	Arranged	Articulated	Ascertained
Asked	Assembled	Assessed	Assigned
Assisted	Assumed	Attained	Attracted
Audited	Augmented	Authored	Authorised
Awarded	Balanced	Began	Benchmarked
Benefited	Bid	Billed	Blocked
Boosted	Borrowed	Bought	Branded
Bridged	Broadened	Brought	Budgeted
Built	Calculated	Canvassed	Captured
Cared	Cast	Catalogued	Categorised
Centralised	Chaired	Challenged	Changed
Channelled	Charged	Charted	Checked
Circulated	Clarified	Classified	Cleared

Closed	Coached	Co-authored	Collaborated
Collected	Combined	Commissioned	Committed
Communicated	compared	Compiled	Completed
Complied	Composed	Computed	Conceived
Conceptualised	Condensed	Conducted	Conserved
Consolidated	Constructed	Consulted	Contacted
Contributed	Controlled	Converted	Conveyed
Convinced	Coordinated	Copyrighted	Corrected
Corresponded	Counselled	Created	Critiqued
Cultivated	Customised	Cut	Dealt
Debated	Debugged	Decentralised	Decreased
Deferred	Defined	Delegated	Delivered
Demonstrated	Depreciated	Described	Designated
Designed	Detected	Determined	Developed
Devised	Diagnosed	Directed	Discovered
Dispatched	Dissembled	Distinguished	Distributed
Diversified	Divested	Documented	Doubled
Drove	Earned	Eased	Edited
Educated	Effected	Elicited	Eliminated
Emphasised	Empowered	Enabled	Encouraged
Endorsed	Enforced	Engaged	Engineered
Enhanced	Enlarged	Enlisted	Enriched
Ensured	Escalated	Established	Estimated
Evaluated	Examined	Exceeded	Exchanged
Executed	Exempted	Expanded	Expedited
Experienced	Explained	Explored	Exposed
Extended	Extracted	Fabricated	Facilitated
Fashioned	Fielded	Financed	Fired
Flagged	Focused	Forecasted	Formalised
Formatted	Formed	Formulated	Fortified
Founded	Fulfilled	Furnished	Furthered
Gained	Gathered	Gauged	Generated
Governed	Graded	Granted	Greeted
Grouped	Guided	Handled	Headed
Helped	Hired	Hosted	Identified
Ignited	Illuminated	Illustrated	Impacted
Implemented	Improved	Improvised	Inaugurated

Incorporated	Increased	Incurred	Individualised
Indoctrinated	Induced	Influenced	Initiated
Innovated	Inquired	Inspected	Inspired
Installed	Instigated	Instilled	Instituted
Instructed	Insured	Integrated	Interacted
Interpreted	Intervened	Interviewed	Introduced
Invented	Inventoried	Invested	Investigated
Invited	Involved	Isolated	Issued
Joined	Judged	Justified	Kept
Launched	Lectured	Led	Lightened
Liquidated	Litigated	Lobbied	Localised
Located	Logged	Maintained	Managed
Manufactured	Mapped	Marketed	Maximised
Measured	Mediated	Mentored	Merchandised
Merged	Minimised	Modelled	Moderated
Modernised	Modified	Monitored	Motivated
Moved	Multiplied	Named	Narrated
Navigated	Negotiated	Netted	Noticed
Nourished	Nursed	Nurtured	Observed
Obtained	Offered	Opened	Operated
Orchestrated	Ordered	Organised	Oriented
Originated	Overhauled	Oversaw	Participated
Patented	Patterned	Performed	Persuaded
Phased	Photographed	Pinpointed	Pioneered
Placed	Planned	Polled	Posted
Prepared	Presented	Preserved	Presided
Prevented	Processed	Procured	Produced
Proficient	Profiled	Programmed	Projected
Promoted	Prompted	Proposed	Prospected
Proved	Provided	Publicised	Published
Purchased	Pursued	Qualified	Quantified
Quoted	Raised	Ranked	Rated
Received	Recognised	Recommended	Reconciled
Recorded	Recovered	Recruited	Rectified
Redesigned	Reduced	Referred	Refined
Regained	Registered	Regulated	Rehabilitated
Reinforced	Reinstated	Rejected	Remedied

Remodelled	Renegotiated	Reorganised	Repaired
Replaced	Reported	Represented	Rescued
Researched	Resolved	Responded	Restored
Restructured	Resulted	Retained	Retrieved
Revamped	Revealed	Reversed	Reviewed
Revised	Revitalised	Rewarded	Safeguarded
Salvaged	Saved	Scheduled	Screened
Secured	Segmented	Selected	Separated
Served	Serviced	Settled	Shaped
Shortened	Shrank	Signed	Simplified
Simulated	Sold	Solicited	Solved
Spearheaded	Specialised	Specified	Speculated
Spoke	Spread	Stabilised	Staffed
Staged	Standardised	Steered	Stimulated
Strategised	Streamlined	Strengthened	Stressed
Structured	Studied	Submitted	Substantiated
Substituted	Suggested	Superseded	Supervised
Supplied	Supported	Surpassed	Surveyed
Synchronised	Systematised	Tabulated	Tailored
Targeted	Taught	Tested	Tightened
Took	Traced	Tracked	Traded
Trained	Transacted	Transcribed	Transferred
Transformed	Translated	Transmitted	Transported
Treated	Tripled	Troubleshot	Tutored
Uncovered	Underlined	Undertook	Unearthed
Unified	United	Updated	Upgraded
Urged	Used	Utilised	Validated
Valued	Verbalised	Verified	Viewed
Visited	Visualised	Voiced	Volunteered
Weathered	Weighed	Welcomed	Widened
Withstood	Witnessed	Won	Worked
Wrote	Yielded		

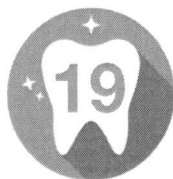

Reference websites

DH (Department of Health)
www.doh.gov.uk

NHS
www.nhs.uk

General Dental Council (GDC)
https://www.gdc-uk.org

National Institute for Health and Care Excellence (NICE)
www.nice.org.uk

Committee of Postgraduate Dental Deans (COPDEND)
https://www.copdend.org

National Advice Centre for Postgraduate Dental Education (NACPDE)
https://www.rcseng.ac.uk/dental-faculties/fds/nacpde/contact-the-nacpde/

Practitioner Performance Advice
https://resolution.nhs.uk/services/practitioner-performance-advice/

ROYAL COLLEGES AND FACULTIES

Faculty of General Dental Practice (FGDP), Royal College of Surgeons of England
https://www.fgdp.org.uk

Faculty of Dental Surgery (FDS), Royal College of Surgeons of England
https://www.rcseng.ac.uk/dental-faculties/fds/

Faculty of Dental Surgery, Royal College of Surgeons of Edinburgh
https://www.rcsed.ac.uk/faculties/faculty-of-dental-surgery

Faculty of Dental Surgery, Royal College of Physicians and Surgeons of Glasgow
https://rcpsg.ac.uk/dentistry/home

Faculty of Dentistry, Royal College of Surgeons of Ireland
https://facultyofdentistry.ie

PROFESSIONAL ASSOCIATIONS

British Society of Paediatric Dentistry (BSPD)
https://www.bspd.co.uk

British Association of Oral Surgeons (BAOS)
https://www.baos.org.uk

British Dental Association (BDA)
https://bda.org

British Association of Oral and Maxillofacial Surgeons (BAOMS)
https://www.baoms.org.uk

British & Irish Society for Oral Medicine (BISOM)
https://bisom.org.uk

British Society for Oral and Maxillofacial Pathology (BSOMP)
https://www.bsomp.org.uk

British Orthodontic Society (BOS)
https://www.bos.org.uk

British Society for Restorative Dentistry (BSRD)
https://www.bsrd.org.uk/Index.aspx

British Society for Periodontology (BSP)
http://www.bsperio.org.uk

British Society of Dental and Maxillofacial Radiology (BSDMFR)
https://www.bsdmfr.org.uk

British Association for the Study of Community Dentistry (BASCD)
http://www.bascd.org

DEANERIES

NORTH
North East (including North Cumbria)
https://madeinheene.hee.nhs.uk/

North West
https://www.nwpgmd.nhs.uk/

Yorkshire and the Humber
https://www.yorksandhumberdeanery.nhs.uk/

MIDLANDS AND EAST
East Midlands
https://www.eastmidlandsdeanery.nhs.uk/

West Midlands
https://www.westmidlandsdeanery.nhs.uk/

East of England
https://heeoe.hee.nhs.uk/

SOUTH
Kent, Surrey and Sussex
https://ksseducation.hee.nhs.uk/

South West: Peninsula Region
http://www.peninsuladeanery.nhs.uk/

South West: Severn Region
http://www.severndeanery.nhs.uk/

Thames Valley
http://www.oxforddeanery.nhs.uk/

Wessex
http://www.wessexdeanery.nhs.uk/

LONDON
https://www.lpmde.ac.uk/

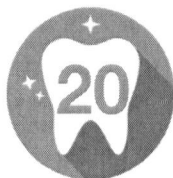

20 Key documents

Standards for the Dental Team

Available from the GDC's website at www.gdc-uk.org

Other guidance documents available from the GDC include:

Guidance on advertising
Guidance on child protection and vulnerable adults
Guidance on commissioning and manufacturing dental appliances
Guidance on indemnity
Guidance on prescribing medicines
Guidance on reporting criminal proceedings
Guidance on using social media
Position statement on tooth whitening
Industrial action guidance
Duty of candour guidance
Mandatory reporting on female genital mutilation (FGM)

Specialist societies may also have a wealth of information on their websites. As an example, the British Society of Paediatric Dentistry (BSPD) has published position papers on infant feeding (2018), obesity and dental decay in children (2015) and water fluoridation (2019). They also have guidelines on areas as diverse as non-pharmacological behaviour management (revised 2011) and clinical holding during dental care of children (2016).

Make sure you access the websites of the professional societies for the specialties you are applying to. The content is often topical and concise, and the documents contained represent valuable resources.

FULL INDEX
OF QUESTIONS
AND ISSUES